WITHDRAWN
UTSA LIBRARIES

D1603683

PSYCHIATRIC CARE
OF MIGRANTS:
A CLINICAL GUIDE

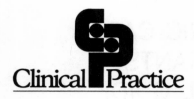

Clinical Practice

Number 10

Judith H. Gold, M.D., F.R.C.P.(C)
Series Editor

PSYCHIATRIC CARE
OF MIGRANTS:
A CLINICAL GUIDE

JOSEPH WESTERMEYER, M.D., M.P.H., Ph.D.
*Professor of Psychiatry and Adjunct Professor of Anthropology
and Psychology, University of Minnesota, Minneapolis,
Minnesota; and Consultant, World Health Organization*

American
Psychiatric
Press, Inc.   1400 K Street, N.W.
Washington, DC 20005

Note: The authors have worked to ensure that all information in this book concerning drug dosages, schedules, and routes of administration is accurate as of the time of publication and consistent with standards set by the U.S. Food and Drug Administration and the general medical community. As medical research and practice advance, however, therapeutic standards may change. For this reason and because human and mechanical errors sometimes occur, we recommend that readers follow the advice of a physician who is directly involved in their care or the care of a member of their family.

Books published by the American Psychiatric Press, Inc., represent the views and opinions of the individual authors and do not necessarily represent the policies and opinions of the Press or the American Psychiatric Association.

Copyright © 1989 American Psychiatric Press, Inc.
ALL RIGHTS RESERVED
Manufactured in the United States of America
First Edition

91   90   89   4   3   2   1

The paper used in this publication meets the minimum requirements of the American National Standard for Information Sciences—Permanence of Paper for Printed Library Materials, ANSI Z39.48-1984.   ∞

Library of Congress Cataloging-in-Publication Data

Westermeyer, Joseph, 1937–
    Psychiatric care of migrants : a clinical guide / Joseph
Westermeyer. — 1st ed.
        p.   cm. — (Clinical practice : no. 10)
    Includes bibliographies.
    ISBN 0-88048-175-7
    1. Immigrants—Mental health. 2. Aliens—Mental health.
3. Psychotherapy. I. Title. II. Series.
    [DNLM: 1. Mental Disorders—therapy. 2. Transients and
Migrants—psychology. WA 305 W527p]
RC451.4.E45W47   1989
616.89—dc19
DNLM/DLC
for Library of Congress   89-412
                                                            CIP

Contents

Acknowledgments

Although I had hoped eventually to write such a book (in the vague and distant future), the actual impetus came from Dr. Judith Gold's work with a migrant patient in her practice. In conversations with colleagues, she found that other psychiatrists shared her dilemmas in caring for this growing group of patients. I am pleased that this book had its inception in such a clinical context, growing out of a current and widespread clinical need rather than just out of my need to formulate a guide for care of migrant patients—long a special interest of mine.

Several psychiatrists have stimulated my interests and influenced my ideas in this field of psychiatry. Among them are Drs. Armando Favazza, Edward Foulks, David Kinzie, James Shore, John Spiegel, Wen-Shing Tseng, Ron Wintrob, and Joe Yamamoto. The recent works of psychiatrists Drs. Edvard Hauff, Keh Ming Lin, Steven Moffic, and Dale Walker have also enriched this work. Critical to the foundation and later evolution of these perspectives on migration and identity have been a score of social science colleagues, among whom are Professors Linda Bennett and John Berry. I am also especially grateful for the insights gained from psychologist James

Butcher, Ph.D., and social worker David Kruzich, D.S.W. Colleagues who have been migrants themselves and who have labored with me in the care and study of migrants have been a rich source of information, encouragement, and energy. They include Dr. Touxa Lyfoung, Ms. Laura Lam, Ms. Mayka Bouafuely, Mr. Geu Vang, and Mr. John Neider.

Personal relationships over the last half century have no doubt driven my fascination with this topic and have fleshed out migration as a lived and shared experience. These relations consist especially of the following: my immigrant grandparents from County Mayo, Ireland, Ellen Roach and Michael McDonagh, with whom I spent many rich days in my childhood; my mother who (with us children) followed my father about the United States during his years of military service in World War II; my wife Rachel and our two children who accompanied me to work in Asia several times; foreign student and "fictive" daughter Chao Xiong Beeson of Laos; and our foster children Meng, Cheng, Kong, Pong, and Pakou Her (children of our departed friends Tou Her and Youa Lo, refugees from Laos). Among other migrant friends and co-workers I want especially to thank Larry Berger, Phikhun and Adul Keomahathai, Dr. Karen Olness, and Hakan Torjesen—survivors themselves of such experiences as the Peace Corps, concentration camp, refugee flight, war, and serving refugees.

Two people are due my special gratitude in bringing this volume to fruition in less than a year. Ms. Gloria Wolf prepared the manuscript and its revisions against stringent deadlines. Michelle Westermeyer diligently searched out hundreds of reference reports, monographs, and books, some of them harbored away in nooks and crannies seldom frequented.

Last and most important, I wish to thank my patients and survey subjects. Their successes and tribulations, struggles and achievements, joys and anguishes—along with their patience and tolerance in ameliorating my ignorance—have largely shaped this work.

Introduction
to the Clinical Practice Series

*O*ver the years of its existence the series of monographs entitled *Clinical Insights* gradually became focused on providing current, factual, and theoretical material of interest to the clinician working outside of a hospital setting. To reflect this orientation, the name of the Series has been changed to *Clinical Practice.*

The Clinical Practice Series will provide readers with books that give the mental health clinician a practical clinical approach to a variety of psychiatric problems. These books will provide up-to-date literature reviews and emphasize the most recent treatment methods. Thus, the publications in the Series will interest clinicians working both in psychiatry and in the other mental health professions.

Each year a number of books will be published dealing with all aspects of clinical practice. In addition, from time to time when appropriate, the publications may be revised and updated. Thus, the Series will provide quick access to relevant and important areas of psychiatric practice. Some books in the Series will be authored by a person considered to be an expert in that particular area; others will be edited by such an expert who will also draw together other knowledgeable authors to produce a comprehensive overview of that topic.

Some of the books in the Clinical Practice Series will have their foundation in presentations at an annual meeting of the American Psychiatric Association. All will contain the most recently available information on the subjects discussed. Theoretical and scientific data will be applied to clinical situations, and case illustrations will be utilized in order to make the material even more relevant for the practitioner. Thus, the Clinical Practice Series should provide educational reading in a compact format especially written for the mental health clinician–psychiatrist.

Judith H. Gold, M.D., F.R.C.P.(C)
Series Editor,
Clinical Practice Series

Preface

*T*his book has been prepared for psychiatrists who treat migrant patients. Other physicians might find the first four chapters of interest, although the last four chapters assume considerable psychiatric knowledge and experience on the part of the reader. Psychiatric nurses and psychologists should have little difficulty comprehending most of the book, with the exception of Chapter 6 on somatotherapies. Social and behavioral scientists interested in migration may utilize Chapters 2 through 5 as overview papers but will certainly want to pursue the original literature via the references. Administrators, planners, and educators may find Chapters 2, 3, and 8 useful.

The book has been organized such that a reading from front to back follows a logical progression. Experienced clinicians can manage it on their own. Residents and graduate students would best read it as part of a seminar or discussion group.

Chapter 1
Introduction

Chapter 1

Introduction

Rationale for this Book

The United States is largely a country of migrants, beginning with the Asian peoples who traveled the Bering Straits land bridge to North America. Post-Columbian centuries brought Europeans and Africans, many of whom have retained distinctive ethnic characteristics. During the twentieth century, migrants have come from Eastern Europe, Latin America, Africa, and South and Southeastern Asia. Temporary migrants to the United States have included students, visitors, diplomats, seasonal workers, and legal and illegal workers. Within our own national boundaries people migrate because of work, education, marriage, or personal preference.

The number of migrants in the United States is impressive. Over a 40-year period in the mid-1900s, 60 million Americans migrated from rural to urban areas while 29 million Americans migrated from urban to rural areas (Hamilton 1965). An estimated 3 million illegal aliens now reside in the United States, many of whom are eligible for citizenship under the new migration law of 1986 (Crockcroft 1986). Approximately 1% of the American population today is composed of refugees. These include 800,000 Cubans, 600,000 Indochinese, and several hundred thousand Europeans since World War II from such countries as Germany, Hungary, Czechoslovakia, Poland, and the USSR (Loescher and Scanlan 1986). Legal immigration continues, adding to the American foreign migrant pool: 601,516 immigrants entered the United States during 1987, probably a higher figure than for all other countries in the world combined (Bacon 1988). A recent economic study group has proclaimed, "America's biggest import is people" (Oxford Analytica 1986). Moreover, the numbers from census data are increasing: from a foreign-born population of 9.6 million in 1970 to 13.9 million in 1980, a 45% increase over one decade (Briggs 1987). The composition of immigrants has changed in recent years from its previous predominance of Europeans. For example, there are about 1 million immigrants from India and about 1 million immigrants from Africa now in the United States.

Refugee movements have also been momentous: 8 million in Europe after World War II, 13 million worldwide in 1979 (Grant 1979), and 16 million worldwide in 1981 (Cohon 1981). A United Nations report estimated that 45 million people had been driven from their homelands from 1945 to 1967 (United Nations 1969). Predictably, refugees and migrants are focused in particular areas. For example, 5.2 million Afghanistan refugees live in Iran and Pakistan, 1.3 to 2.0 million refugees in East Africa, and about 500,000 refugees in Southeast Asia (Chanda 1988). By the year 2000, 750,000 South Asians will be resident in Canada (Buchignani et al. 1985). Other forms of migration have also been massive. Turkish workers in Germany and Sweden, Algerian workers in France, Portuguese workers in Switzerland, Thai workers in the Middle East, Korean workers in Africa, and other migrant workers number in the millions (Chaney 1986). Over 100,000 illegal aliens in Japan alone have fled economic stagnation in South Asia and Africa (Hamilton 1965). Returning military compose another large group counted in the millions.

Migration to and within the United States will continue actively in the foreseeable future. Countries of Europe and Asia, now experiencing social, political, and economic problems with asylum-seekers, are restricting entry (Billard 1985; Jefferson 1988), with resultant pressure on the United States to increase its refugee and immigrant quotas. Opposition to more immigration has been due to the drain on public services by legal and illegal immigrants (in excess of tax revenues generated by immigrants), to opposition by organized labor, and to high welfare and disability rates among some immigrant groups (Briggs 1987; Hammond 1988; Muller and Espenshade 1985).

Psychiatrists and Migrants

Migrants often contribute much to their new communities. Hard work, entrepreneurial spirit, academic achievement, a labor pool for industry, and other advantages have been well described (Herbst 1988; Jefferson 1988). Migrants also pose special psychiatric problems for clinicians, as well as for society at large. Migration can precipitate psychiatric disorder, exacerbate it, and, in some unusual cases, relieve it. Understanding migration as a pathogenic factor can provide the clinician with enhanced understanding of patients' disorders and offer insights into alleviation of these disorders.

Psychiatrists generally recognize the importance of sociocultural factors in the care of patients, at least on a theoretical level. On a practical level, however, many of us have little awareness of our own sociocultural attitudes, values, and the culture-bound attributes of psychiatric practice itself (Moffic and Adams 1983; Wintrob and Youngsook 1981). Even when aware of general sociocultural factors in a given patient, psychiatrists may not know how to use this awareness in the service of the patient (Kleinman 1977). This problem has been considered over the last several years by the American Psychiatric Association, the American Association of Directors of Residency Training in Psychiatry, and several academic psychiatrists (Foulks 1980; Moffic and Adams 1983; Moffic et al. 1987; Yager 1982). Despite increasing recognition of the importance of this area in psychiatric practice, residency education on minority and sociocultural issues actually declined from the 1970s to the 1980s (Moffic et al. 1987). A recent study of psychiatric diagnoses of Cuban refugees in the United States has demonstrated the poor diagnostic reliability when psychiatrists untrained in cross-cultural diagnosis assess migrants (Boxer and Garvey 1985).

Purpose and Organization

The primary goal of this book is to improve the psychiatric care of the migrant patient. To accomplish this, the clinician must possess background information regarding types of migration and their normal processes (Chapter 2). Discussion of psychopathology among migrants (Chapter 3) alerts the clinician to the common psychiatric manifestations in migrants. Clinicians must have conceptual tools at hand to aid in the assessment of the migrant patient (Chapter 4). The second half of the book (Chapters 5 to 8) covers therapeutic as well as public health interventions. These chapters assume training and experience in medicine and psychiatry, so that only special issues relevant to various migrant patients are addressed. Topics include special issues and principles of clinical management, pharmacotherapy and other somatotherapies, psychotherapies, hospitalization, and various sociotherapies (including social readaptation and acculturation therapies).

References

Bacon KH: Population and power: preparing for change. Wall Street Journal 69(164):1 (June 6), 1988

Billard A: China: keep the birth rate down! Refugees 17:31–32, 1985

Boxer PA, Garvey JT: Psychiatric diagnoses of Cuban refugees in the United States: findings of medical review boards. Am J Psychiatry 142:86–89, 1985

Briggs VM: The growth and composition of the U.S. labor force. Science 238:176–180, 1987

Buchignani N, Indra DM, Srivastiva R: Continuous Journey: A Social History of South Asians in Canada. Toronto, McClelland-Stewart, 1985

Chanda N: Questions of quotas. Far Eastern Economic Review, Vol 140, April 7, 1988, pp 30–32

Chaney R: Regional Emigration and Remittances in Developing Countries: The Portuguese Experience. New York, Praeger, 1986

Cohon JD: Psychological adaptation and dysfunction among refugees. International Migration Review 15:255–275, 1981

Crockcroft JD: Outlaws in the Promised Land. New York, Grove Press, 1986

Foulks EF: The concept of culture in psychiatric residency education. Am J Psychiatry 137:811–816, 1980

Grant B: The Boat People: An "Age" Investigation. New York, Penguin Books, 1979

Hamilton HC: Educational selectivity of migration from farm to urban, and to other non-farm communities, in Mobility and Mental Health. Edited by Kantor MB. Springfield, IL, Charles C Thomas, 1965

Hammond R: Strangers in a strange land: Minnesota's troubled Hmong. Twin Cities Reader, June 7, 1988, pp 1–10

Herbst J: Migration helps poorest of the poor. Wall Street Journal 69(169):22, (June 15) 1988

Jefferson DJ: Land of opportunity. Wall Street Journal 69(164):26R–31R (June 10) 1988

Kleinman AM: Rethinking the social and cultural context of psychopathology and psychiatric care, in Renewal in Psychiatry: A Critical Rational Perspective. Edited by Kleinman AM, Manscherk TC. New York, Wiley, 1977, pp 97–138

Loescher G, Scanlan JA: Calculated Kindness: Refugees and America's Half-Open Door, 1945 to the Present. New York, Free Press, 1986

Moffic HS, Adams GL (eds): The psychiatric care of "minority" groups (special issue). Am J Soc Psychiatry 3:10–24, 1983

Moffic HS, Kendrick EA, Lomax JW, et al: Education in cultural psychiatry in the United States. Transcultural Psychiatric Research Review 24:167–187, 1987

Muller T, Espenshade TJ: The Fourth Wave: California's Newest Immigrants. Washington, DC, Urban Institute, 1985

Oxford Analytica: America in Perspective. Boston, Houghton
    Mifflin, 1986
United Nations: Refugee Report. Geneva, United Nations High
    Commissioner for Refugees, 1969
Wintrob R, Youngsook KH: The self-awareness factor in inter-
    cultural psychotherapy: some personal reflections, in Coun-
    seling Across Cultures. Edited by Peterson P. Honolulu,
    University of Hawaii Press, 1981, pp 10–132
Yager J: Teaching Psychiatry and Behavioral Science. New
    York, Grune & Stratton, 1982

Chapter 2

Orientation to Migration and Migrants

Chapter 2
Orientation to Migration and Migrants

Definitions and Classifications

For purposes of this book, *migrants* are defined as those who change their place of residence for any purpose or for any period of time. Included are such groups as students going away to school, transferred or migratory workers, people whose work may necessitate travel, tourists, visitors, wanderers, refugees, and those returning home after a migration.

Classifications of migrants have several purposes. Strict legal categories affect the migrant's social rights and privileges in the new place. Other classification systems are based on the characteristics of the migrant, the motivations for the migration, and the duration since relocation or attributes of the migration itself. As we shall see in subsequent sections and chapters, all of these may have mental health implications.

Migration can be categorized according to geographic variables, such as moves from one country to another (Odegaard 1932) or in-country moves (i.e., rural to urban, urban to urban, and urban to rural). Relocations may involve ethnic change, such as a Native American (e.g., American Indian, Eskimo, Native Hawaiian) from a traditional community seeking training or work in a city.

Certain occupations may require migration, such as anthropology, diplomacy, higher education, journalism, military service, missionary work, Peace Corps, sales and distribution of certain goods, seasonal migratory work, and the travel industry. Return migrants are those returning home after a period away (Rhoades 1979). Others, such as tourists, are seeking rest or recreation.

Demographic characteristics of individuals and groups have proven significant in understanding the migration experience. Children, adolescents, young adults, the middle-aged, and the elderly experience the changes of migration in different ways, even though they are exposed to similar environmental alterations. Men and women can undergo different modifications in their life-styles and different phases of acculturation (Westermeyer et al. 1984). Education level can weigh heavily in postmigration adjustment. Nor do the effects of migration end with the first generation of migrants themselves. Some evidence indicates that even their children and grandchildren are affected in various ways that may be beneficial as well as detrimental (Leichty 1963; Naditch and Morrissey 1976). Japanese migrants to the United States have labeled their own three generations since migration (i.e., Essei, Neisei, Sansei) based on their differing characteristics.

Migrants have been categorized on the voluntariness of their relocation (Berry et al. 1987). Governments have forced their citizens to relocate for such reasons as construction of dams, roads, and other projects; and testing of military equipment (Fahim 1983). Refugees fleeing from prejudice and persecution would generally prefer to remain at home but feel forced to leave the homeland. Prisoners of war must involuntarily adjust to a new culture from the unique setting of incarceration; failure to adjust appropriately can be lethal. Those in prison for committing crimes must adjust to a new residence and life-style, albeit in their own culture (unless incarcerated abroad). Foster children and those placed in remedial juvenile institutions must accommodate while also dealing with loss and behavioral or mental-emotional problems. Workers may be forced to relocate from depressed economic regions to seek work. Some communities in the United States must literally export their youth in order to remain economically viable (Mayer and Ahern 1969). Family members may willingly relocate with a wage earner, although preferring to remain in place. To a greater or lesser extent, these travelers are pushed out of their homes, rather than pulled or drawn to a new location (Kunz 1981). Resettlers or guest workers may pursue social or economic advantages elsewhere merely because they are not available at home. Many migrants go entirely willingly to the new place, for example, most tourists, missionaries, Peace Corps workers, and members of the diplomatic corps.

Duration of the relocation is often an important variable in ascertaining the phase of readjustment as well as the likelihood of social maladaptation or psychiatric disorder. Time spans under consideration may be only hours or days in the case of tourists, or years or decades in the case of refugees. There may be two "durations" for refugees—that since leaving the home country and that since arriving in the resettlement country. The temporal intent of the migrant may be to relocate permanently to a new home, or to relocate temporarily for a specific time span (e.g., 2 weeks of vacation, a season of harvesting, 2 years of military service overseas, 4 years of college). The relocation pattern may become one of episodic relocation, such as the schedule of a seasonal migratory worker or the diplomat reassigned from one country to another.

Vintages of migrants have been described (Kunz 1981). For example, the first wave of recent Southeast Asian refugees has primarily had more education, more occupational skills, more exposure to complex society, and more previous affiliation with Americans (Stein 1979; Westermeyer et al. 1983) compared with later refugees, who have come primarily for economic reasons or to reunite the family. Later waves have typically required more social support, training, and education than earlier groups.

Migrants have been compared on the basis of cultural similarity and/or dissimilarity (sometimes referred to as "cultural distance") between the culture of origin and the culture of resettlement (Berry et al. 1987). Some relocations involve extensive linguistic, ecological, political, technological, social, and family change (e.g., an unaccompanied adolescent refugee from Asia or Africa in the United States). Other migrations involve little sociocultural change, but sudden and dramatic changes in social network and life-style (e.g., a new soldier in boot camp, a New Yorker going off alone to a small rural Midwestern college). Geographic distance can also affect the migrant's ability to satisfy emotional needs by returning home at intervals. For example, a newly married man joining his wife in Minneapolis has easier access to his relatives if the latter live in Chicago rather than in Australia.

Presence and extent of victimization have been assessed in migrants, beginning with refugees and prisoners of war from World War II. Away from their sources of security and initially unaware of means for assuring their own safety, migrants are at risk to victimization. Terrorist and kidnap victims also have to cope with threat and removal from familiar surroundings and people. In flight, and even initially during resettlement, refugees are at risk to assault, murder, rape, theft, and burglary. Combat veterans have had to cope with loss under circumstances that rarely permit adequate grief work.

Governmental determinations are important factors in working with migrants. Each foreign migrant with a passport and visa has a specific legal status, with highly regulated restrictions, rights, and obligations. These affect such elements as duration of stay in the country, legal rights, social privileges, and access to special government-supported programs. Recently these regulations have been changed and will probably undergo further modifications in future years. Information on the current regulations can be obtained from a regional office of the Immigration and Naturalization Service (INS). Federal immigrant visa categories include tourist, visitor, student, worker, refugee, and immigrant. Currently there are over 1 million illegal migrants in the United States (and probably as many as 3 million). Governmental status may not resemble the actual psychosocial characteristics of a given migrant. For example, some immigrants or illegal migrants may in fact be fleeing persecution (and thus meet United Nations criteria for refugee status) but be from a friendly country so that refugee status is not legally feasible. Or some legal status "refugees," especially from later waves or "vintages," may not meet United Nations criteria but wish to relocate to get out of a war-torn or civil-strife area, to meet personal financial ambitions, or to rejoin an extended family. State or provincial regulations may affect clinical care under certain situations. For example, refugees from a given state may not be eligible for care in another state unless the state of residence authorizes care (which they are usually reluctant to do because of revenue loss to another state).

Changes Associated with Migration

Travel over several time zones disturbs various circadian rhythms, a condition known colloquially as "jet lag." In addition to transient sleep loss and sleep disturbance, other bodily functions that vary around the clock are also altered for some days or weeks. Endocrine functions, most of which vary around the clock, may contribute to psychiatric disorder. Elderly people, those with chronic medical conditions, and former psychiatric patients are especially vulnerable in the early postmigration period (Streltzer 1979).

Ecological changes can be disturbing, especially when a large difference exists between the new and old residence. Unfamiliar topography, climate, housing style, modes of transportation, and neighborhood—perhaps quaint during a brief visit—can be unsettling when one must fit into them. It may be necessary to change clothing styles and diet. Even personal grooming may need to change due to climate, local custom, or unavailability of familiar grooming aids.

Migrants often complain that the new population distribution is too dense or too sparse, depending on their past exposure and preference. Racial and ethnic gaps may exist between the former and present home, so that someone accustomed to being in the majority may assume minority status (or vice versa). Migrants may encounter racial or ethnic prejudice for the first time.

Language and communication present major obstacles in migration across countries or from one ethnic community to another. Acquisition of a limited number of everyday expressions and the ability to shop and travel can take several weeks to several months, depending on one's ability and devotion to the language-learning task. Children and adolescents may be reasonably fluent at the end of 1 year in a new country, while young adults often require 2 years for good language skills (Krupinski and Burrows 1986). Middle-aged migrants may never reach social fluency but can usually attain adequate language for work and ordinary social functions. Elderly migrants often do not reach a level adequate even for self-sufficiency in a new language. Languages, like cultures, have smaller or larger "gaps." It is easier to learn a new Romance or German or Slavic language if one already knows another one. Tonal languages initially are particularly difficult for non-tonal speakers, and vice versa. Regional dialects and idiomatic speech are further complications.

Communication involves more than language. Newcomers must learn dimensions of nonverbal communication, such as appropriate distance between speakers, eye contact, physical touch, local forms of gesticulation, and means of expressing emotion. Using humor in interpersonal relationships, asserting oneself to another, expressing displeasure or frustration, requesting a favor, or initiating pre-courting communication all require an advanced degree of communication skill. Without these skills the migrants live in a kind of social isolation, unable to perceive others' feelings or to express their own. This emotional isolation can be a pathogenic factor, especially in migrants without access to a family or expatriate community.

Social network loss is an almost inevitable concomitant of migration. Forced relocations or refugee moves can result in the movement of an entire intact community to a new location so that social network loss is minimized (Fahim 1983; Westermeyer 1985). The solitary migrant is at increased risk to a variety of mental health disorders (Gordon 1964; Walsh and Walsh 1987; Westermeyer and Berger 1977). Access to both family and friends in the new environment is ideal. For those going into a new cultural setting, access to an expatriate community can be crucial in maintaining links to the familiar past. Isolation within family and an expatriate community can also lead to problems by prolonging, delaying, or blocking adjustment to the new society, thereby fostering cultural isolation.

Vocational changes are a component of many migrations. Even those continuing in the same vocation must adjust to new co-workers, an unfamiliar work environment, and new challenges. Relocation, even with the same employer, typically involves changes in role, responsibilities, work task, and resources to meet the demands. Refugees and guest workers must adjust to the new occupational and employment realities of the host society (Finnan 1982). Migrating students encounter new teaching styles and teachers' expectations.

Avocations, hobbies, sports, or other recreational activities rarely can be continued unchanged. Some activities are not feasible due to climate, local resources, or regulations. These losses can be great for those whose self-identities are strongly linked to these pastimes. Development of skill at new pastimes requires time, energy, and material resources—scarce commodities for many migrants. Several years often pass before new avocations replace lost ones.

Social roles, along with their special status and prestige, are ordinarily left behind in the old community. New associates do not know or, perhaps more to the point, do not care if one was formerly the class president, a village headman, a skilled sportsman, a devoted daughter, a decorated soldier— or other role with no currency in the new society. One must struggle anew to establish a social identity that is personally comfortable and appreciated by others. This subtle and difficult process requires years, even decades.

Loyalties to the past conflict with loyalties in the present. Some of these are mundane and of no great consequence (e.g., which sports team to support). Others are more substantial. Balancing important commitments to the past and present involves decisions regarding time, money, and other resources. One must be favored at a cost to the other, or both must be compromised. Migrants can end up disappointing, even alienating associates from the past. Adaptation to current realities may result in feelings of disloyalty to old commitments. If national loyalties are involved, the personal struggles can be deep and prolonged.

Religious practice may or may not pose a problem, depending on the resident's religious commitments and the relocation community. Dietary restrictions, special religious grooming or dress, and need for a group of fellow believers can create problems for staunch or fundamentalist practitioners. Local moral standards or even certain government regulations can create severe conflicts.

Laws, regulations, and legal status in the new community are disruptive to many migrants. Lawful behaviors in the old society, such as polygamy or severe physical punishment of children, can lead to serious legal consequences. Regulations of the INS, if not strictly adhered to by foreign migrants, can result in sudden expulsion. Those accustomed to full citizen status in their own country may feel personally diminished by their noncitizen "guest" status in the new country.

As sojourners become familiar with the new language and acquire social networks in the new society, they encounter differences in the attitudes, values, beliefs, and mores. These may be minimal and easily worked through or so drastic as to demand a total reorientation of the self—a difficult and risky proposition, a virtual revolution of the self. On the political level, many refugees represent political extremes that resulted in their expulsion or flight. Royalists, elitists, socialists, communists, anarchists, and others may be strongly disenchanted with the local political climate.

Developmental changes that vary across the life cycle can precipitate problems in the family migrating across cultural boundaries. Experiences in the new society affect people at different ages in such diverse ways that intergenerational conflict is an inevitable aspect of family relocation. Older family members recoiling against certain aspects of the new society find their own younger family manifesting these very characteristics. As a result of their more rapid language acquisition and entry into the local culture, children may serve as translators and socializers for their parents and grandparents—a potentially stressful role reversal for all concerned. Spouses often find fundamental changes occurring in their marital relationship. Men may be unable to find employment, and women may have to enter the workplace. As a defense against these unsettling family conflicts, the family (or at least its older members) may retreat to an ethnic enclave.

Permanent resettlers are often surprised to encounter delayed culture conflicts throughout their lifetimes, even after they have made adjustments that are successful on a day-to-day basis. Crises occur in certain predictable patterns. One problem is the life event in which the familiar patterns of the old culture are replaced by those of the new society. Examples include a new job, marriage, childbirth, medical care and hospitalization, legal problems and court proceedings, parenting and relationships with schools, death, and funeral practices. Another problem occurs when other family members behave in ways discordant with the traditional culture but in ways acceptable in the United States. Common examples include children questioning or disagreeing with parents, and a family member marrying outside the ethnic group. An Asian father committed suicide when his adult son, using his own earnings, purchased a car without the father's consent. An Asian mother attempted suicide when her teenage daughter brought home a male schoolmate to meet her parents without first arranging the meeting with both sets of parents. These crises, stemming from cultural conflicts and losses of one kind or another, can reawaken earlier conflicts and losses. Refugees in particular may experience depression, posttraumatic stress symptoms, and other disorders after decades of interim successful adjustment. Retirement or the death of a spouse may precipitate such problems even decades after migration.

Returning home after months or years away is often considered a joyful event rather than a stressful migratory event. Several factors can contribute to a problematic reentry, however. Homeward travelers have usually changed as a result of age and life experiences or education during their interim away. If they have made a successful adjustment to a setting markedly different from their home communities, they are somewhat different individuals from those who originally left home. This change can create dilemmas for the migrants as well as their relatives and former associates. The kin group and community will also have changed in various ways over a period of years, necessitating reentry to an altered setting (Wintrob 1967; Rhoades 1979; Guendelman and Perez-Itriago 1987).

Rationales for Migrating

One of the prime reasons for migration, whether in-country or international, is seeking or continuing work (Applebaum 1966). Employment opportunities may be sparse in rural areas, small towns, some metropolitan areas, many resort communities, and American Indian reservations (Mayer and Ahern 1969). Massive legal and illegal migrations are rooted in the underemployment and poverty of certain regions. National and international corporations expect certain categories of workers to relocate. Certain occupations require migration repeatedly throughout a career. Certain occupations are favored in particular locales, such as art colonies near vacation areas or publishing companies in New York. Often advancement or promotion in one's vocation demands one or more career migrations.

Business opportunities in the United States motivate more immigration than is generally appreciated. A little-known fact is that foreign business people with large sums of money may receive special visas as a means of correcting the balance of payments and stimulating commerce with other countries and within the United States. This quiet "money migration" wave, mostly from South and East Asia, has gone heavily into the food and lodging industry.

Education and training stimulate much relocation. Education of thousands of foreign students has become a growth industry for many North American and European colleges and universities. Most of the students come from developing countries or smaller countries. Thousands of American students also return home each year from education abroad.

Migration fosters more migration through marriage of partners from different regions. People often travel during early adult years when courting occurs. Marriages between young people with limited education and cross-cultural experience often do not fare well. The immigrant spouses of these unions are at high risk to require psychiatric services. A small but increasing clinical problem consists of indigenous spouses whose foreign spouses have married to obtain a permanent resident visa. Once aware of the actual situation, the indigenous spouse is at risk to psychiatric disorder.

Kunz (1981) has described two kinds of refugees based on identity and reasons for migrating: (1) "majority identified" nationalists who reluctantly flee due to imminent charges from the government or a foreign oppressor and then long to return home, and (2) "events alienated" marginal or minority persons who, alienated by rejection or persecution, flee rapidly to seek new opportunities and identities. Examples of the former are Ukrainian, Chilean, and Lao refugees. Examples of the latter are the Chinese refugees out of Vietnam, Hmong refugees out of Laos, and Indian refugees out of Uganda. By international convention, flight from war or civil strife does not qualify for refugee status, but nonetheless several hundreds of thousands of migrants have fled to North America legally or illegally to escape conflicts in Latin America, Africa, and Asia. Disaster victims from floods, tornadoes, dams breaking, ground pollution, and atomic energy accidents also experience dislocations along with property loss and sometimes loss of life. Removal for public purposes (e.g., water reservoirs, mining, roads) also involves a forced migration.

Brief travel can permit a time-out from one's usual roles and responsibilities. Erikson (1956) has referred to this as a "psychosocial moratorium" when it is undertaken out of uncertainty and dissatisfaction in order to reassess one's life, chart new paths, and set new goals. Smith (1966) has identified this motivation as a major factor in Peace Corps volunteers. Student travel can meet education goals in ways not feasible in the classroom (e.g., language training, practicums, internships). Retreats for work, study, research, or religious purposes permit participants to inundate themselves in a project or undertaking not possible in ordinary life. Honeymoons often involve travel away from family and friends, allowing the couple a period of adjustment to each other and to their new relationship. Travel is not a prerequisite for such time out from social obligations, but it does facilitate the process by removing one from the workplace, household duties, the telephone, reciprocal obligations to friends and family, and the other chores of daily life.

Psychological factors such as boredom, the desire for a new social identity, a devastating failure, divorce, or death of a spouse can precipitate migration. Milestones in life, such as graduation, marriage, or retirement, also provide an occasion for changing one's residence. A potential problem lies in the fact that, of themselves, these psychological rationales may involve a reason for leaving a place but not necessarily a reason for going to a particular place. Those migrants are sometimes referred to as escapists. As Jensen (1966) has observed, self-serving or impulsive escapism may prevail even among those with other valid rationales to relocate, including refugees. Altruistic motivations (e.g., among missionaries, foreign aid workers), while not explicitly self-serving, still contribute to enhanced self-esteem. Carried to an extreme, altruistic impulses can lead to messianic expectations, which are then frustrated, leading to a sense of failure. Returning students can also suffer the consequences of their messianic anticipations after returning (Wintrob 1967). Like the lead character in *Portnoy's Complaint,* some people unable to achieve sexual gratification near home may need to travel a distance in order to express their sexuality (Frosch and Auchincloss 1981).

Pathological reasons for migration may exist. In Hawaii, the "coconuts and bananas syndrome" refers to migrants who come expecting that life is simple and easy, with food readily available from nearby trees and unoccupied grass huts awaiting them on the beach (Streltzer 1979). Those migrating because of loneliness or alienation are apt to rediscover loneliness or alienation in their new location. Those with a major depression may erroneously expect that travel will reverse the disorder. A substance abuser may seek to escape alcohol or drugs by the well-known "geographic cure." Psychotic persons may migrate for psychotic reasons. "Cargo cult" movements— first described in Oceania (Burton-Bradley 1975)—have occurred several times over the last few decades in the United States, with several thousand people gathering at a specific location to await preternatural largesse or the end of the world. Chronically unhappy persons may become habituated to travel as a means of temporarily relieving their ennui, until dysthymia stimulates another cycle of travel. Refugees may harbor expectations of a politico-military reversal so they may return to familiar roles and life-styles—a possibility that rarely occurs. This lingering hope for a triumphant return can undermine adjustment in a foreign land.

The reasons for moving to a new place are often not the same reasons for remaining in a place. Rationales thus change over time. Often several reasons for remaining coexist, some of which may even seem mutually incompatible or contradictory. Clinically, it is helpful to understand the individual's rationales for migrating and for remaining. No one-to-one relationship exists between the migration rationales and the clinical consequences. Those moving for the most well considered factors can still encounter psychiatric disability. Conversely, escapists can reintegrate and find a comfortable and productive niche in the new locale.

Biopsychosocial Processes of Migration

Travel across several time zones can affect menstrual cycles for a few to several months. Mittelschmerz may occur. Disturbed sleep functions begin returning to normal within days but may require several weeks to return to normal.

Local water supply and diet can also create gastroenteric disturbances. Abdominal and bowel symptoms may persist for days or weeks. Stool cultures, stool for ova and parasites, and gastrointestinal consultation should be obtained if symptoms persist.

Extensive travel and relocation stress can exacerbate numerous medical conditions, including the following: hypertension and cardiac conditions; eczema, asthma, hay fever; malaria, amebiasis, enteric parasites; psoriasis, rheumatoid arthritis; hypothyroidism, hyperthyroidism, diabetes. Some of these conditions may mimic psychiatric disorders.

"Culture shock" has been used to label the common psychological experiences of those adapting to a new culture (Garza-Guerrero 1974). An initial touristic phase consists of curiosity with the new environment; bemusement with or interest in unfamiliar dress, customs, or topography; superficial perceptions and analyses of events; and a detached acceptance toward the local people. After some weeks, the sojourner enters a phase of disconsolation with the current location, loneliness, and thoughts of home. The imperfections of the local society loom greater in the person's awareness, while the defects of the former setting recede from consciousness. If the obsessional longing for the past residence is severe, sufferers may refer to this state as homesickness. Several alternatives are available at this point. The individual may return home (not possible for most refugees or military personnel), stay and try to accommodate to the new community (perhaps the most difficult option), or cling to a local enclave of like persons (thereby accepting a marginal status in the new place). If the migrant chooses accommodation, special efforts are needed over a period of months and years.

Certain types of migrants may have additional emotional tasks during this period of social readjustment. Refugees, forced resettlers, and victims of natural disasters need to grieve their losses (Baskauskas 1981). Grief work demands time, energy, and a degree of security that the victim may not possess in the midst of dealing with harsh realities. Delayed or missed grief associated with various psychiatric disorders may ensue. Prolonged residence in refugee camps and other types of relocation camps over months or years can create a state of resentful apathy and dependence (Bakis 1955; Pfister-Ammende 1973). These personality traits can become permanent features.

Adjustment styles can alter the subjective experience and the observable behavior of a migrant during adjustment. Meszaros (1961) has described the following reaction types:

- Over accepting: enthusiastic, denies difficulties, struggles to adapt to the new situation, suppresses hostility, may reject own former ethnic identity;
- Actively critical: rejects new setting, makes unfavorable comparisons, idealizes former community, depressed, feels discriminated against;
- Inhibited: emotionally withdrawn, expresses little feeling toward past or present environment, may be insecure or fearful;
- Hyporeactive: perplexed, feels lost, unable to undertake readjustment tasks, dissatisfied, bitter, chronically lonely, homesick;
- Hyperreactive: emotionally labile, alternating behavior patterns, may become violent or otherwise act out, is at risk to brief psychosis or suicide attempt.

Berry (1976) has discerned three migrant adjustment styles, which may apply either to individuals or to groups, as follows:

- Adjustment: the conflicts resolved by trying to make the two cultural or regional backgrounds more similar or integrated (i.e., movement toward);
- Reaction: attempts to reduce the conflict by retaliating against the source of the conflict, such as by political organization (i.e., movement against);
- Withdrawal: the conflict is abandoned by returning home or entering an ethnic enclave (i.e., movement away).

Khoa and VanDeusen (1981) have described three adjustment patterns:

- Old line pattern: rejection of the new culture, refusal to adapt, manifested mostly by elderly people;
- Assimilative pattern: embracing the new customs and giving up the old, manifested mostly by the young;
- Bicultural pattern: selectively adapting new customs while maintaining some former ones.

Lin et al. (1982) have posited five alternative routes for coping with cultural changes induced by migration:

- Neurotic marginality: develops high levels of anxiety while trying to comply with expectations of both cultures;
- Deviant marginality: becomes isolated due to ignoring norms of both cultures after being unable to satisfy both simultaneously;
- Traditionalism: withdraws into the old culture to escape loss and confusion;
- Over-acculturation: abandons the former culture, loses traditional supports, more vulnerable;
- Biculturation: integrating both cultures with the best possible compromises.

Four basic forces that drive the migrant's adjustment can be discerned. One factor is the migrant's personality, which can determine the attitude toward the change and the course chosen to deal with the change. A second factor is the degree of difference or similarity between the migrant's previous "donor community" and the new "receiver community." A third factor is the attitude of the receiver community toward the migrant. A fourth factor is age, with older people leaning toward the traditional past, younger people reaching for the future, and adults dealing with the bicultural present.

Ensocialization consists of the training and education of citizens from birth in the skills, knowledge, attitudes, values, and mores of their society. Without thorough grounding as a child, adults cannot fully acquire the cultural accoutrements gained through the ensocialization of the infant, child, and adolescent by the family and the community. The earlier the exposure to another society, the more complete the ensocialization process. Living in the home of an indigenous person, working in the local community, or marrying a local person facilitates greater ensocialization than might otherwise occur during adulthood. Learning the local language is critical for greater ensocialization to occur. Adult migrants, deprived of ensocialization during childhood, cannot encounter the experiences available to children. The gap in the ensocialization of migrant parents (in the previous culture) and their migrant children (in the new culture) accounts for much of the intergenerational gap observed in these families.

Acculturation refers to the changes in cultural patterns when two different cultural groups have ongoing contact with one another. Although both groups might change as a result of the contact, in fact the dominant group ordinarily produces more changes in the weaker group. The dominant group is usually larger, occupied the locale first, and/or has more political and economic power compared with the weaker group. This process of acculturation occurs via the psychological and social processes described in this section (Chance 1965).

Cultural competence refers to the ability of people to function effectively and efficiently in a culture at a level consistent with their own goals and social roles. The language and social competence required for a young working person differs from that of a retired person. The level of survival skills for a 2-week vacation in a country lies below those needed for a 2-year work assignment. The cultural knowledge and social skill expected of a foreign-born psychiatrist greatly exceeds that of a foreign-born physicist. Cultural competence is strongly tied to language ability, awareness of the prevailing norms and mores, and skill in accomplishing necessary tasks.

The acculturative process can have several outcomes, depending on the individual's efforts and goals, and the intercultural relationship existing between the migrant group and the receiving group. Assimilation occurs when a separate social and cultural identity ends, and the nondominant group is absorbed politically and economically into the societal mainstream. The merging of many groups has been referred to as the "melting pot" phenomenon, in which diverse groups intermarry, live in the same communities, and socialize together (Gordon 1964). Pluralism consists of social integration in the larger society while maintaining distinctive ethnic identities. Diverse ethnic groups share common government, medical and educational institutions, access to financial and corporate entities, and public accommodations such as restaurants and lodging. However, ethnic groups can remain distinctive by conducting their own worship, celebrating their own annual events, conducting their own family rituals, inducing their young to marry into the group, forming their own social organizations, and retaining their own customs and cultural identity (Cavalli-Sforza et al. 1982). This distinctiveness may or may not involve ethnic dress, grooming, language, and other characteristics. Berry (1976) has suggested a category of multiculturalism, in which a pluralistic nation officially supports the notion of a heterogeneous society. Murphy (1986) has posited that migrants to multicultural societies experience less stress and better mental health compared with migrants going to unicultural societies.

Migrants sometimes form an ethnic enclave in which all or most people in a neighborhood, village, or town belong to the same cultural group. This strategy enables the group to maintain traditional language, dress, social norms, and other cultural attributes. In the short run, these ethnic enclaves provide a familiar and supportive environment for the migrant. Over the long run, they can maintain a marginal or subcultural status, which delays acculturation and impedes the migrant's entry into the political and economic mainstream. Such enclaves can run afoul of the majority society by engaging in traditional but illegal practices, such as polygamy, family-forced marriage, bride kidnap, gang wars, drug production and commerce, or revenge murders. It is of course possible to have a supportive expatriate community that is still involved in the social mainstream. Such a group can contribute considerably to the acculturation process by providing time-out respite from the adaptive efforts. Members can also help in acculturating one another and by sharing their experiences, frustrations, and successes. Vicarious learning in the expatriate group greatly enlarges members' knowledge, as well as giving members support to attempt new behaviors and take risks. Expatriate communities can provide entrees to work, economic opportunities, and new friends (Bar-Yosef 1968).

Anomie, the abandonment of cultural norms and values, poses serious social and psychiatric risks. Harsh imposition of the dominant culture and suppression of the indigenous culture can produce this result. A classic example is the treatment accorded American Indians in the United States, who were forbidden for decades to conduct their traditional ceremonies or to speak their own language.

Research in several cultures has demonstrated the strong association of social network size with mental health (Cassel 1974; Cobb 1976; Tran 1987; Westermeyer and Pattison 1981). Most functional adults report 20–30 people in their intimate social network. Larger networks require too much time and effort to maintain, since these relationships involve regular contacts and interdependence. Relationships between the proband and the network members are reciprocal. Psychiatric patients and chronically ill people tend to have small networks of 10–19 people, with asymmetric reciprocity. Psychiatric inpatients and those living in institutions tend to be locked into a single subgroup of fewer than 10 people. Migrants, whether students or refugees, become involved in reestablishing a normal-sized social network, having usually lost members as a result of the migration.

The process of social network reconstruction proceeds normally when there are others nearby who are similarly involved with expanding their networks (e.g., college freshmen or military inductees at boot camp). This process does not proceed easily if one is the only recent arrival among others who already have a surfeit of network obligations. Examples include an immigrant spouse coming to a new community, a refugee family placed away from other refugees, or a housewife involuntarily relocated to a new community because of her husband's job transfer. Social network reconstruction in these latter cases can be long and tedious, requiring many friendly overtures and repeated disappointments until a congenial set of new associates is acquired. Organizations that require episodic relocation often hold "newcomer" rituals to facilitate this process. For example, the military, the diplomatic corps, academic institutions, and retirement communities have special social gatherings for this purpose.

Characteristics of the receiving community have major effects on postmigration adaptation. If the receiving community views the migrants as taking hard-to-find jobs, occupying sparse housing, reducing their own access to social and medical services, and imposing a new cultural standard, conflicts are inevitable. Such situations can become dangerous for both migrants and receiving-community members. In other instances, the host community welcomes and facilitates the newcomer (Finnan 1982).

Characteristics of the migrant group can also affect the adaptive outcome (Kleis 1981). For example, early Cuban migrants from the 1950s and 1960s did well in the United States, whereas those released from Cuban prisons and mental institutions who arrived in 1980 have had a high rate of institutionalization in the United States. Prolonged dependency in refugee camps tends to have adverse consequences (Pfister-Ammende 1973). A "colonial mentality" among Filipino immigrants to the United States has been said to limit their adaptive capacity (Lott 1976). The rationale for the migration can also influence the severity of the subjective stress reported by migrants (Berry et al. 1987).

Historical Aspects of Migration and Psychiatry

An estimated 37 million people came, escaped to or were kidnapped into this country during the 150 years following the Declaration of Independence (Dawes 1924–25). The first concerns about mental disorder among migrants to the United States began in the 1820s and 1830s. During this period several countries of Europe paid for transport of prisoners, mentally retarded, mentally ill, and impoverished persons to the United States. For example, the British government appropriated grants and loans between 1834 and 1886 to send 40,000 paupers, insane, and chronically diseased persons to the United States. A Congressional committee considered the problem in 1838. The hearings and resultant legislative recommendations were sufficient to reverse temporarily the European penchant for solving their local mental health problems by forced emigration to the United States. The problem recurred in the 1850s, when several European countries were found to be pardoning murderers if they would emigrate to the United States. Again congressional inquiries and foreign diplomacy worked for a time. When abusive emigration recurred, the first of a series of immigration laws was promulgated in 1882, followed by further restrictions in 1891, 1903, 1907, and 1971 (May 1907; Dawes 1924–25).

Special Logistical Considerations

Reduction in or absence of the social network can compromise clinical assessment as well as treatment. Collateral information, often critical in assessing premorbid function and recent stressors, may be limited in the migrant patient. Assistance with socialization, physical mobilization, monitoring medication and vegetative signs, and other clinical assistance may not be available. Hospitalization or residential treatment can be indicated in the absence of an adequate social network.

If the patient is unfamiliar with English or another language known to the clinician, a translator must assist with assessment and treatment. The need to wait for translations in both directions more than doubles the time required for communication. Both the presence of a second person (the translator) and the need for extra time can double or even triple the cost of assessment and care.

If the patient comes from a cultural group with which the psychiatrist is not familiar, this also adds to the time required for assessment and care. Background information on the culture, extra facilitation and clarification to avoid misunderstandings, and more education of the patient are usually necessary. A "cultural consultant" (e.g., a countryman of the patient, an anthropologist, or other person familiar with the culture) may be needed.

The patient's or family's view of the mental disorder may differ greatly from that of the clinician (Guilmet and Whited 1987; Clement 1982). As with indigenous patients, it is important to understand their view of the malady and its management in order to negotiate, educate, and improve treatment compliance. Notions regarding confidentiality, the locus of control of the individual vis-à-vis society, attitudes toward autonomy and responsibility, theoretical views on the origins of mental abnormalities, and other relevant concepts are often critical to compliance, treatment, and outcome (White and Marsella 1982). Family structure and problem solving can differ widely (Dunnigan 1982).

All societies have culturally influenced modes for signaling distress. Most of these modes are common to all societies (e.g., suicide attempt), but the distribution varies from one culture to the next. Some presentations are extremely rare in some societies while being relatively more frequent in others, for example, anthropophobia, latah, amok, anorexia, bulimia, substance abuse (Friedman and Faguet 1982).

Literacy cannot be assumed with many migrants from developing regions. Evaluating the illiterate patient presents special challenges, since few Western psychiatrists have extensive experience with illiterate people nowadays. The illiterate person may have a high intelligence or be retarded. Psychological assessments may be difficult because testing relies heavily on literacy. Another problem is the post-infancy onset of mental retardation—an infrequent problem in the United States, but not unusual in migrant children exposed to later brain insults from infection, malnutrition, or trauma. These patients may be literate or socially skilled on a superficial level, but have severe intellectual deficits.

At times our diagnostic nomenclature fails us in dealing with the migrant patient. Chronic adjustment symptoms, persisting over years or decades, are encountered, although our American Psychiatric Association Diagnostic and Statistical Manual, Third Edition and Revised Third Edition (DSM-III and DSM-III-R), require that symptoms clear in weeks to qualify for an adjustment reaction. Some of these patients have symptoms in minor depression or anxiety range that were clearly precipitated by migration (Westermeyer 1988).

Financing the psychiatric care and assessment of certain migrant groups presents serious obstacles. Illicit migrants and refugees, tourists, and visitors have no legal access to care in the United States. Students or immigrants may or may not have insurance or adequate personal resources, but overall they have inadequate coverage in the event of a serious psychiatric disorder. Public psychiatric resources are already strained by the demands of indigenous patients on sparse resources, so that special training and staff resources are rarely available.

Private insurance or prepaid programs create obstacles to avoid the extra time and expense necessary for translation, special consultation, and the extra time needed for assessment and care. Hopefully these impediments to care will dissolve as psychiatric leaders and planners become educated to the special needs of the migrant patient.

References

Applebaum RP: Seasonal migration in San Ildefonso Ixtahuacan: its causes and consequences. Public and International Affairs 4:117–158, 1966

Bakis E: D.P. apathy, in Flight and Resettlement. Edited by Murphy HBM. Paris, UNESCO, 1955

Bar-Yosef RW: Desocialization and resocialization: the adjustment process of immigrants. International Migration Review 2:27–45, 1968

Baskauskas L: The Lithuanian refugee experience and grief. International Migration Review 15:276–291, 1981

Berry JW: Human Ecology and Cognitive Styles: Comparative Studies in Cultural and Psychological Adaptation. New York, Sage-Halstead, 1976

Berry JW, Kim V, Minde T, et al: Comparative studies of acculturative stress. International Migration Review 21:491–511, 1987

Burton-Bradley BG: Stone Age Crisis: A Psychiatric Appraisal. Nashville, TN, Vanderbilt University Press, 1975

Cassel J: Psychological process and "stress": theoretical formulation. Int J Health Serv 4:471–482, 1974

Cavalli-Sforza LL, Feldman MW, Chen KH, et al: Theory and observation in cultural transmission. Science 218:19–27, 1982

Chance NA: Acculturation, self-identification, and personality adjustment. American Anthropologist 67:372–393, 1965

Clement DC: Samoan folk knowledge of mental disorders, in Cultural Conceptions of Mental Health and Therapy. Edited by Marsella AJ, White GM. Dordrecht; Boston: D. Reidel; M.A. Hingham, 1982, pp 193–213

Cobb S: Social support as a moderator of life stress. Psychosom Med 38:300–314, 1976

Dawes SL: Immigration and the problem of the alien insane. Am J Psychiatry 4:449–470, 1924–25

Dunnigan T: Segmentary kinship in an urban society: the Hmong of St. Paul-Minneapolis. Anthropologist Quarterly 55:126–134, 1982

Erikson EH: The problem of ego identity. J Am Psychoanal Assoc 4:56–121, 1956

Fahim HM: Egyptian Nubians: Resettlement and Years of Coping. Salt Lake City, University of Utah Press, 1983

Finnan CR: Community influences on the occupational adjustment of Vietnamese refugees. Anthropological Quarterly 55:161–169, 1982

Friedman CTH, Faguet RA: Extraordinary Disorders of Human Behavior. New York, Plenum, 1982

Frosch WA, Auchincloss EL: Geographic reinforcement of the incest taboo: three case vignettes. Am J Psychiatry 138:679–680, 1981

Garza-Guerrero AC: Culture shock: its mourning and the vicissitudes of identity. J Am Psychoanal Assoc 22:408–429, 1974

Gordon MM: Assimilation in American Life: The Role of Race, Religion and National Origins. New York, Oxford University Press, 1964

Guendelman S, Perez-Itriago A: Migration tradeoffs: men's experiences with seasonal lifestyles. International Migration Review 21:709–727, 1987

Guilmet GM, Whited DL: Cultural lessons for clinical mental health practice: the Puyallup tribal community. American Indian and Alaska Native Mental Health Research 1:32–49, 1987

Jensen FAS: Psychological aspects of the social isolation of refugees. International Migration Review Digest 3:48–51, 1966

Khoa LX, VanDeusen JM: Social and cultural customs: their contribution to resettlement. Journal of Refugee Resettlement 1:48–51, 1981

Kleis GW: Comparative perspectives on migrant adaptation: Asian refugees and African sojourners. Journal of Asian African Studies 16:269–275, 1981

Krupinski J, Burrows G: The Price of Freedom: Young Indochinese Refugees in Australia. New York, Pergamon, 1986

Kunz EF: Exile and resettlement: refugee theory. International Migration Review 15:42–51, 1981

Leichty MM: Family attitudes and self concept in Vietnamese and U.S. children. Am J Orthopsychiatry 33:38–50, 1963

Lin KM, Masuda M, Tazuma L: Adaptational problems of Vietnamese refugees, III: case studies in clinic and field—adaptive and maladaptive. Psychiatric Journal of the University of Ottawa 7:173–183, 1982

Lott JT: Migration of a mentality: the Filipino community. Social Casework 57:165–172, 1976

May JV: Immigration as a problem in the state care of the insane. American Journal of Insanity 64:53–71, 1907

Mayer M, Ahern J: Personality and social class position in migration from an island: the implications for psychiatric illness. Int J Soc Psychiatry 15:203–208, 1969

Meszaros AF: Types of displacement reactions among the post revolution Hungarian immigrants. Canadian Psychiatric Association Journal 6:9–19, 1961

Murphy HBM: The mental health impact of British cultural traditions, in Transcultural Psychiatry. Edited by Cox JC. London, Croom Helm, 1986, pp 179–195

Naditch MD, Morrissey RF: Role stress, personality and psychopathology in a group of immigrant adolescents. J Abnorm Psychol 85:113–118, 1976

Odegaard O: Emigration and insanity: a study of mental disease among the Norwegian born population of Minnesota. Acta Psychiatrica et Neurologica Scandinavica Supplement IV, 1932, pp 1–206

Pfister-Ammende M: Mental hygiene in refugee camps, in Uprooting and After. Edited by Zwingmann C, Pfister-Ammende M. New York, Springer-Verlag, 1973

Rhoades R (ed): The Anthropology of Return Migration. Norman, OK, University of Oklahoma Press, 1979

Smith MB: Explorations in competence: a study of Peace Corps teachers in Ghana. Am Psychol 21:555–566, 1966

Stein BN: Occupational adjustment of refugees: the Vietnamese in the United States. International Migration Review 13:25–45, 1979

Streltzer J: Psychiatric emergencies in travelers to Hawaii. Compr Psychiatry 20:463–468, 1979

Tran TV: Ethnic community supports and psychological well-being of Vietnamese refugees. International Migration Review 21:833–841, 1987

Walsh A, Walsh PA: Social support, assimilation, and biological effective blood pressure levels. International Migration Review 21:577–591, 1987

Westermeyer J: Mental health of Southeast Asian refugees: observations over two decades from Laos and the United States, in Southeast Asian Mental Health: Treatment, Prevention, Services, Training and Research. Edited by Cowan TC. Washington, DC, National Institute of Mental Health, 1985, pp 65–69

Westermeyer J: DSM III psychiatric disorders among Hmong refugees in the United States: a point prevalence study. Am J Psychiatry 145:197–202, 1988

Westermeyer J, Berger L: World traveler addicts in Asia, I: demographic and clinical description. Am J Drug Alcohol Abuse 4:495–503, 1977

Westermeyer J, Pattison EM: Social networks and mental illness in a peasant society. Schizophr Bull 7:125–134, 1981

Westermeyer J, Vang TF, Lyfong G: Hmong refugees in Minnesota: characteristics and self perceptions. Minn Med 66:431–439, 1983

Westermeyer J, Bouafuely M, Vang TF: Hmong refugees in

Minnesota: sex roles and mental health. Med Anthropol 8:229–245, 1984

White GM, Marsella AJ: Cultural conceptions in mental health research and practice, in Cultural Conceptions of Mental Health and Therapy. Edited by Marsella AJ, White GM. Boston, D Reidel, 1982, pp 1–38

Wintrob RM: A study of disillusionment: depressive reactions of Liberian students returning from advanced training abroad. Am J Psychiatry 123:1593–1598, 1967

Chapter 3
Psychopathology

Chapter 3
Psychopathology

*M*igrants can suffer any or all of the psychiatric disorders that affect nonmigrants. However, certain disorders are altered or influenced by the migration process. For example, an individual with a chronic mental disorder (e.g., chronic or recurrent psychosis, dysthymia, organic brain syndrome) may have achieved a certain level of coping in the former community but can then become dysfunctional in the new community. Or certain premigration factors (e.g., war experiences, political oppression) or postmigration factors (e.g., loss of social network, racism) may precipitate a psychiatric disorder.

Diagnostic classifications in this chapter are according to the Diagnostic and Statistical Manual of Mental Disorders (DSM-III-R). However, the studies referenced here involve numerous other diagnostic systems, including DSM-I, DSM-II, DSM-III, ICD-8, and ICD-9. Overlap in diagnostic criteria among these systems permits the reader to make informed comparisons if the historical and national differences in diagnostic practice are appreciated.

Psychiatric Emergencies Soon After Migration

Emergency conditions can occur in any type of migrant: tourists and students, immigrants and refugees, wanderers and workers. Bioendocrine stress, premigration vulnerability, and/or unusual stresses typically play a more crucial role than in the later onset cases. Disorders especially frequent in this early phase include acute psychoses, alcohol- and drug-related problems, acute exacerbations of preexisting psychiatric conditions (e.g., schizophrenia), acute anxiety disorders (e.g., panic, social phobia, agoraphobia), and dissociative conditions (Kimura et al. 1975; Streltzer 1979).

A 16-year-old mentally retarded Lao refugee boy was seen for disobedience, oppositional behavior, temper tantrums, destruction of property around the house, and getting lost in the neighborhood. These problems had begun within weeks of arriving in the United States. In Laos, he had assisted family members in their daily chores, functioning well with supervision. In the United States, he was left in the home alone while family members attended school, training courses, and work; he had no responsibilities and was not supervised. The patient responded to placement in a special educational day program, supplemented by a brief course of neuroleptic medication.

Depression

So-called "nostalgia" has long been known among various migrant groups (Rosen 1975). However, early studies of admission for depression to state hospitals did not show inordinate rates among immigrants compared with native-born Americans (Odegaard 1932; Malzberg 1936). Later studies began to show more consistent elevations of state hospital admissions not only for foreign-born individuals, but also for native-born individuals migrating into New York State from elsewhere in the United States (Malzberg 1962, 1964).

Losses associated with forced migration appear particularly apt to precipitate depression in a significant minority of refugees. Among 100 Hmong refugees, 20% were treated in psychiatric settings for major depression over a decade after arriving in the United States (Westermeyer 1988). Depressive conditions appear to be greatest in the early years following relocation, with gradually decreasing rates over time (Koranyi et al. 1963). Social isolation or severe loss of self-esteem, as in the elderly, can produce more severe and longer lasting depression (Ruiz 1982).

Chronic minor depression has also been observed in migrants, especially involuntary migrants such as refugees and concentration camp survivors. This has been referred to variously as dysthymia, depressive neurosis, concentration camp syndrome (Krupinski et al. 1973), immigrant's hypochondriasis (Hes 1958), psychosomatic dysadaptation syndrome (Seguin 1956), and migrant's chronic adjustment disorder (Westermeyer 1988). Many also have symptoms of anxiety, suspiciousness, social withdrawal, and learning inhibition.

Substance Abuse

Early postmigration substance abuse is most commonly observed in business travelers, tourists, and vacationers, rather than permanent resettlers. History, collateral informants, physical examination, and laboratory testing usually suggest a prolonged period of substance abuse that has become worse during the time away from home.

The hospital rates for alcoholic psychosis and other alcohol-related diagnoses have varied with the origins of the migrants (Malzberg 1962; Roberts and Myers 1954). For example, Irish-born migrants in the United States and England have consistently shown increased alcoholism rates compared with local populations (Malzberg 1963; Roberts and Myers 1954; Bagley and Binitie 1970). At the other end of the spectrum, West Indian immigrants in London have shown high rates of psychiatric admission for all other psychiatric disorders, but low rates of admission for alcoholism and drug dependence (Hemsi 1967).

Among migrants from other countries, the substance being abused may be common in that setting but unusual in the United States. Examples include betel-areca dependence (Westermeyer 1982b), and opium abuse and dependence. Substance abuse in migrants often coexists with other psychiatric conditions.

A 36-year-old Hmong widow from Asia presented with opium addiction. Prior to becoming addicted, she had been fearful of the dark and of attending funerals beginning with the death of her 6-year-old daughter 12 years ago in an attack on her village. At the time of presentation she had persisting phobias and panic attacks, along with opium addiction.

Exposure to drug production, smuggling, and selling is another common cause for substance abuse in migrants. Refugees, immigrants, diplomats, returning military personnel and tourists, and other migrants are involved with illicit drug commerce (Westermeyer, 1989). A decrease in learning ability as a result of substance abuse impedes acculturation. Opportunities for illicit wealth, combined with acculturation failure, foster involvement in the drug trade.

Depression, social phobia, agoraphobia, and posttraumatic stress disorder can lead to substance abuse, as migrants attempt to reduce their symptoms by taking alcohol or illicit drugs (Horowitz 1986). Use of nontraditional substances may lead to abuse of new substances. Illicit drug and alcohol abuse has been especially common among younger male refugees (Page et al. 1985; Morgan et al. 1984). This often occurs in association with family disruption, losses, and failure experiences in the new society.

Two teenage boys, Lao refugees, stole money for cannabis and alcohol from their widowed mother. When she confronted them and forbade their stealing, they struck her and threatened her. Resolution of the problem involved treatment for all three family members, with placement of the sons in foster homes for a year.

Paranoia

Anecdotal cases of paranoia have long been reported in guest workers, students, immigrants, and refugees (Edwards 1972; German and Arya 1969; Prange 1959; Tyhurst 1951). Frequency of this disorder in migrants has led to application of special terms such as *aliens' paranoid reaction* (Kino 1951) and *refugee neurosis* with suspiciousness, depression, and somatization (Pedersen 1949). Kendler (1982) demonstrated that immigrant patients, hospitalized in Massachusetts and Michigan, showed a higher rate of paranoid psychosis than locally born patients—a higher ratio, in fact, than for either schizophrenia or affective disorder. Among post World War II displaced persons in Canada, Tyhurst (1954) observed a high rate of suspiciousness and paranoia in patients with all diagnoses. Filipino psychiatric patients in the U.S. Navy displayed paranoid features more often than other Navy patients (Duff and Arthur 1967). West African students hospitalized at the Maudsley and Bethlem Royal Hospitals in England demonstrated prominent paranoid symptoms, especially in association with schizophrenia (Copeland 1968). These reported cases generally involve agitation, depression or hostility, fright and/or assault. Family history of psychosis is typically absent. In the preneuroleptic era, these patients often responded to supportive psychotherapy and electroconvulsive therapy—modalities that infrequently help in paranoia among nonmigrants. These data suggest an affective component in many paranoid cases among migrants. European refugees in England had psychiatric hospitalization for paranoia far more often than native-born patients (Hitch and Rock 1980).

Shared delusional disorder, usually with paranoid components, occurs among socially isolated couples (called *folie à deux*) or families (*folie à famille*). While early observers provided little sociocultural information regarding these cases, Tseng (1969) described a *folie* case in a Taiwan-dwelling refugee family from China. Numerous *folie* cases have been observed among refugees in the United States.

Schizophrenia

In his hallmark work in the 1930s, Odegaard (1932) demonstrated a higher rate of hospitalization for schizophrenia among Norwegian immigrants to Minnesota, using Minnesota-born

Norwegian-Americans and Norwegians in Norway as controls. He also showed that the risk was not simply an early postmigration phenomenon, but continued over many years. Among 344 migrant cases of schizophrenia, 22% of cases began within 5 years of arrival; 27% of cases began 5–10 years after arrival; and 51% of cases began after 10 years following arrival. Rates of hospital admissions per 100,000 per year were 27.9 for Norwegian-born immigrants in Minnesota and 13.8 for Norwegians in Norway. Of interest, Malzberg (1962, 1963) also observed that the crude rate of schizophrenia among foreign-born Irish was 1.8 times higher than the crude rate among native-born Americans; however, the age-adjusted rate comparison was slightly lower than 1.8 times (i.e., 1.5 times). Age at onset of symptoms was the same in both countries, but the average duration of symptoms prior to hospitalization tended to be longer in Minnesota. Salmon (1907) also commented on the apparent delay between onset of symptoms and hospitalization for mentally disordered immigrants. Krupinski (1967) similarly found that care for both depression and alcoholism was delayed for immigrants compared with local people in Australia. I have observed long delays after onset of symptoms (i.e., from several months to several years) before psychotic or severely depressed refugees first enter treatment. Lazarus et al. (1963) found that native-born American migrants in New York, Ohio, and California had higher rates of schizophrenia (adjusted for age) than foreign-born migrants or native-born in-state nonmigrants. When their data were broken down by sex, however, the female foreign-born migrants and the native-born migrants both showed higher schizophrenia rates than the native-born nonmigrant women. Correcting for occupational status, Clark (1948) found higher age-adjusted schizophrenia rates among foreign-born than native-born Chicagoans. Correcting for geographic residence, using 11 different residence zones, Faris and Dunham (1960) observed higher hospitalization rates for schizophrenia among foreign-born compared with native-born Chicagoans. Among a group of Hungarian refugees, paranoid schizophrenia was the most common type, with delusional content being political in nature, such as fear of Communists (Mezey 1960a, 1960b).

Some families from developing countries evidence considerable shame at having a family member with chronic mental illness. The family member may be kept at home for years, until a severely regressed state occurs. The dementia praecox syndrome described prior to social and pharmacological treatment for schizophrenia, still occurs in some migrant groups. Clinical management of these regressed cases is difficult. Family cooperation with treatment may be minimal, and outcome is often poor. Especially in cases with limited acculturation, return to the country of origin can result in a better level of recovery and function.

Mania

Odegaard's study (1932) suggested that mania might be slightly lower in migrants. Malzberg's later work (1936, 1962, 1964) showed slightly higher rates in migrants. However, the data on mania have never been as impressive as those on depression, paranoia, and schizophrenia in migrants. Nonetheless, difficulties can arise in the assessment and treatment of mania in migrants. Due to cultural, ethnic, or regional differences, mania may be mistaken for schizophrenia by clinicians unfamiliar with treating migrants. The clinical picture may also be modified. For example, mania patients from Asia manifest the usual vegetative and psychological symptoms of mania (such as insomnia and racing thoughts), and perhaps certain behaviors such as hypersexuality and pathological gambling, but are less apt to be assaultive, intrusive, and demanding. Migrants with greater acculturation to the United States do demonstrate these latter, more assertive symptoms.

Posttraumatic Stress Disorder

Numerous types of migrants are at risk to posttraumatic stress disorders (PTSDs). These include returning veterans and prisoners of war, concentration camp internees, survivors of disasters, and refugees. Symptoms of PTSD include nightmares and/or intrusive thoughts of the traumatic event, feelings of guilt or shame, fatigue, anergy, somatization, problems acquiring new information (e.g., language, job training), and minor symptoms of anxiety and/or depression (Chodoff 1963; Ostwald and Bittner 1968). When present alone (i.e., without other psychiatric disorder), these disorders often resolve by themselves over a period of weeks or months.

Most PTSD cases that bring migrants to clinical attention involve an associated psychiatric condition. By far the most commonly associated disorder is major depression. Other associated conditions include phobias, generalized anxiety, and panic attacks. Especially in victims of torture, war injuries, and other physical mistreatment, organic brain syndrome may also be present. Current losses or stresses may precipitate PTSD even years or decades after the traumatic events. Precipitating events include not only job loss, but also death in the family, theft or burglary, retirement, and similar losses or threats to security (e.g., vandalism). The traumatic event may happen during the postmigration phase, rather than before migration. The absence of a social network in the new setting may result in more psychopathology than might otherwise be the case. Tyhurst (1951) reported that among World War II refugees, "all patients" had such recurring nightmares and dreams. While that statement cannot be applied to all refugees, still such experiences occur in many refugees and other victims of violence. If other Axis I diagnosis is absent, occasional PTSD symptoms may be bothersome but are rarely disabling. Often they show a tendency to wane with time, but may return if another psychiatric condition develops.

Somatization

The categories listed above are considered disorders. Somatization, a symptom rather than a disorder, consists of the somatic expression of psychosocial distress. Pain complaints may focus in any anatomic distribution, but are often manifest as headache, backache, or abdominal pain. Other symptoms include those that accompany anxiety and depression: fatigue, anergy, constipation, diarrhea, feeling hot or cold, palpitation, tachycardia, dyspnea, tachypnea, dry mouth, paresthesias, lightheadedness, clouding of consciousness, urinary frequency, epigastric distress, scotomata, tinnitus, tremor, and similar psychophysiological symptoms. Somatization may occur in various psychiatric conditions, from adjustment disorders to major depression, psychotic depression, panic disorder, generalized anxiety, the phobic disorders, organic brain syndrome, and somatoform disorder.

Migrants from postwar Europe in Tyhurst's Canadian study (1951) were often referred to her psychiatric clinic for somatic complaints. A decade later, Mezey (1960a) observed that about one-half of 82 Hungarian refugees presented with somatic symptoms at a British psychiatric facility. Nguyen (1982) has remarked on the regrettable practice of extensive laboratory investigations in refugees with depression and anxiety. In a group of 250 refugees seen in our psychiatric clinic, presenting complaints fell into the following categories: 50% somatic complaints, 29% psychosocial complaints, 11% somatic plus psychosocial complaints, and 10% other complaints (e.g., forensic referrals). Those patients presenting with somatic complaints were more apt to be older, unemployed, less educated, and suffering an anxiety-phobic-panic or depressive disorder compared with those presenting with psychosocial complaints. While these patients volunteered somatic symptoms, they were willing to acknowledge psychological symptoms when asked about them. Italian migrants to Australia have also been prone to somatization (Pasquarelli 1966). Other migrants have also shown tendencies toward somatization (Hull 1979).

Somatization among migrants may be due to several factors. Migrants may come from cultures that discourage direct emotional expression, while favoring somatic expressions of anxiety, depression, and other psychiatric maladies. It may be more comfortable for migrants to express somatic rather than psychological distress to strangers. Those migrants who have had to stifle their emotions to survive (e.g., veterans, prisoners of war, refugees) may be less attuned to the psychological symptoms of psychiatric disorder while perceiving the somatic symptoms (Lin et al. 1985). Migrants often experience stress-precipitated psychophysiological disorders such as atrial tachycardia, allergic rhinitis (hay fever), asthma, eczema, hives, rheumatoid arthralgia, and migraine.

Schizophreniform or Brief Reactive Psychosis

Acute psychoses have often been reported in migrants undergoing considerable stress in a context of social or cultural isolation (Eitinger 1959; Lin et al. 1982). Ordinarily there has been no premorbid disability nor family history of psychosis. Symptoms may be florid, with hallucinations, delusions, and confusion. Paranoid symptoms are usually present and may predominate in migrants, making the clinical picture similar to a paranoid psychosis. Affective symptoms (depressive or manic) also occur to a greater or lesser extent. Spontaneous resolution or response to brief low-dose neuroleptic medication help to establish the diagnosis.

Organic Brain Syndrome

International migration consists heavily of persons from developing countries going to industrialized countries. Due to generally poorer health conditions in the former countries, migrants are more exposed to infectious disease and malnutrition that may affect the central nervous system (CNS). Migrants from rural to urban areas in many developing countries are also at risk to CNS damage. Brain trauma must also be considered in returning veterans, prisoners of war, refugees, concentration camp survivors, torture victims, political prisoners, and other potential victims of violence.

Thiamine deficiency as well as pellagra can account for CNS damage in migrants. Infectious diseases producing chronic

CNS impairment in migrants include encephalitis (e.g., mumps, measles), meningitis (e.g., pneumococcal, tuberculous), and certain parasitic diseases (e.g., malaria). Damage from prolonged dehydration, heat exhaustion, heatstroke, high fever, and untreated status epilepticus have also been observed. Physical abuse methods causing brain damage consist of beating about the head, inundation of the head in water or other fluid (e.g., petroleum products, mud, urine), and other modes of oxygen deprivation (e.g., occlusion of mouth and nose, plastic bag over head).

Acquired Mental Retardation, Learning Disorders, and Attention Deficit Disorder

Migrant children, adolescents, and adults are apt to present with cognitive and learning disabilities that differ from those ordinarily encountered in nonmigrants. Etiological factors are largely those accounting for organic brain syndrome in adults. However, the interaction between child development and brain insult, preinsult and postinsult educational experiences, and nature of associated ensocialization-acculturation experiences do produce unusual clinical pictures that warrant special consideration in migrants (Williams and Westermeyer 1983). Some disorders that have not been encountered for decades in some industrialized countries, such as cretinism, still occur in migrant groups.

Mental retardation in developed countries has generally been present from birth or infancy in most cases. Elsewhere mental retardation frequently begins during childhood or even early adolescence. Retention of earlier social and intellectual skills may persist, although the person's ability to acquire new information or solve problems is compromised. Consequently, the patient may appear to be more competent than is the actual case.

Migrants are apt to acquire learning disabilities later in childhood, or even in adulthood. These can seriously impede the migrant's ability to learn a new language in the resettlement country. Attention deficit disorder (ADD) can be difficult to recognize in migrants, especially if hyperactivity is not present.

Culture-Related Syndromes

Migrants infrequently present with syndromes that, although common enough in the culture of origin, may be extremely rare in the psychiatrist's culture. In the past these were sometimes referred to as culture-bound disorders, although the work of Simons and Hughes (1985) and others (Friedman and Faguet 1982) has shown that these syndromes are collections of well-known psychiatric signs and symptoms that can occur virtually anywhere (e.g., amok or berserk, latah, koro, arctic hysteria, spirit possession). Anxiety and behavioral components weigh heavily in these syndromes, whose rates vary greatly from one culture to another. Clinicians sometimes assume that the syndromes compose a distinct psychiatric disorder, when in fact they do rarely, if ever. Complete psychiatric assessment is needed in order to make a diagnosis, create a treatment plan, and set a prognosis. The syndromes may herald problems ranging from adjustment disorder to psychosis.

A 33-year-old migrant from Asia complained that his penis and testicles were shrinking into his abdomen (i.e., the koro syndrome), causing fatigue, insomnia, and weight loss, and possibly his imminent death. Medical examination and extensive laboratory tests elsewhere had failed to alleviate his concern. He observed his penis disappearing and his testicles bulging up under the skin of his thighs and abdomen. Tricyclic medication relieved the vegetative symptoms of his major depression; neuroleptic medication was eventually required to alleviate his somatic hallucinations and delusions. Recovery was gradual over a several month period.

These folk syndromes are similar to American folk syndromes such as "nervous breakdown" or "cardiac neurosis." For example, the clinician must determine whether the patient is fearful of developing or dying of a heart disease or is convinced that the heart has died or death is imminent. Over time there is a tendency for migrants to develop the culture-related syndromes manifested by the people among whom they live (Westermeyer 1982a). This phenomenon is further evidence of the pathoplastic nature of certain psychopathology.

Missed, Complicated, or Delayed Bereavement

Migrants encounter this problem more frequently than do others. Some migrants, such as tourists, guest workers, or students, are away from home when a death or other loss occurs. Absence of this sort may prevent their engaging in necessary grieving with those who also experience the loss. Returning veterans and refugees sometimes sustain losses under conditions that are not conducive to normal grieving (e.g., prolonged combat or threat). Torture victims, those in exile, or other migrant victims also experience losses that require grief work in order to move on into the future.

A 42-year-old refugee with major depression had recurrent nightmares regarding his mother. During flight she had become ill and weak. He carried her for 2 days, until she asked to be left behind. For the survival of his family and the rest of the group, they could not remain with her. During the subsequent weeks and months, the flight and adjustments in the refugee camp did not permit grief work, and the family did not have a corpse as a central feature for traditional grieving. In treatment, as he was responding to tricyclic medication, grief work was initiated.

Senility

Displacement of the elderly to new circumstances can severely compromise their former adjustment. Loss of familiar routines, separation from an established social network, and the need to learn a new geographic situation can produce stress, depression, and confusion. Chronic biomedical conditions can become worse, further exacerbating mental and emotional function. Assessment requires careful medical as well as psychiatric evaluation.

> A 72-year-old Vietnamese widow was brought to the United States by her family. Her chronic diabetes and hypertension became worse and she became confused. She remained awake much of the night, cooking inedible meals and exhausting the family's food supply. She also hid her family's clothing around the house. Depressive symptoms became more prominent as the patient's medical problems were controlled. Her inappropriate behavior and depression responded to family intervention, socialization with other elderly Asians, and tricyclic medication.

Violence, Pathological Gambling, Sociopathy

Certain migrant groups, composed mostly of young males, can be at risk to antisocial behaviors dangerous to society (King and Locke 1987). The thousands of criminals, delinquents, and psychiatrically ill persons sent by the Cuban government to the United States during the Mariel boatlift can be seen as one blatant example. This tragedy, which has led to the murder of scores of people, many hundreds of expensive court cases, and thousands of crimes in the United States, remains unresolved as of this writing. Hungarian refugees from the uprising in that country also created numerous violent disturbances in Europe and North America (Koranyi et al. 1963; Mezey 1960b; Meszaros 1961). Unaccompanied refugee children and adolescents may have had to survive on their own by stealing, prostitution, or other illegal activities; they are a group at high risk, often for a prolonged period (Tans 1983). The nature of sociopathic expression can vary among cultures.

> A 56-year-old Asian woman came to live with her daughter and American son-in-law. The precipitant for the move was discord with her husband, as a result of which he had taken a minor wife. As she had done before in times of stress, the

woman ran up a gambling bill of several thousand dollars. She also showed symptoms of an adjustment reaction with minor depressive symptoms.

Physical Disorders Complicated by Psychological Factors

Numerous physical conditions can precipitate psychiatric disorders. Or conversely, psychological factors can exacerbate physical conditions. Such problems are frequent in migrants. The clinician must be alert to conditions that occur infrequently in native-born patients but are more common in certain migrants. These include the following:

- Neoplasms: craniopharyngioma, hepatoma, choriocarcinoma;
- Infectious disease: tuberculosis, schistosomiasis, amebiasis, leprosy;
- Endocrine abnormalities: thyroid inflammation, hyperthyroidism;
- Certain congenital disorders: hemoglobinopathies from malarious regions.

Epidemic Psychiatric Disorders

Isolated migrant groups can develop delusional systems, often with a paranoid component. In one refugee family with a shared delusional disorder, a mass suicide attempt took place, led by the psychotically depressed father. A mentally ill religious leader in Jonestown, Guyana, led several hundred Americans in a mass suicide. Social isolation, internal group discord, and mentally deranged leadership can result in these dangerous outcomes.

A classic example of an epidemic fixed belief was the kachigami delusion among tens of thousands of Japanese immigrants in Brazil after World War II. Those affected by this delusion insisted that the Japanese Empire had won the war. They aggressively opposed anyone, especially Japanese, who denied victory. Severe disruption broke out in the Brazilian Japanese community. Over 15 community leaders were assassinated, and discord affected the community for several years after World War II. As in other community examples, there was a combination of isolation of the Japanese community from other Brazilians as well as severe internal dissonance between traditional and modern views within the Japanese community.

Delusions of parasitosis or other infectious disease (e.g., venereal disease) may be isolated to individuals, or they may spread *folie*-fashion within families, clans, or portions of communities. Failure of acculturation, low education, unemployment, and internal family or community strife are again common associated themes. Major depression occurs in a large percentage of those with the epidemic form of this disorder, unlike the paranoid syndromes observed in isolated cases.

References

Bagley C, Binitie A: Alcoholism and schizophrenia in Irishmen in London. Br J Addict 65:3–7, 1970

Chodoff P: Late effects of the concentration camp syndrome. Arch Gen Psychiatry 8:323–333, 1963

Clark RE: The relation of schizophrenia to occupational income and occupational prestige. American Sociological Review 13:325–330, 1948

Copeland JRM: Aspects of mental illness in West African students. Soc Psychiatry 3:7–13, 1968

Duff DF, Arthur RJ: Between two worlds: Filipinos in the U.S. Navy. Am J Psychiatry 123:836–843, 1967

Edwards AT: Paranoid reactions. Med J Aust 1:778–779, 1972

Eitinger L: The incidence of mental disease among refugees in Norway. J Mental Science 105:326–328, 1959

Faris REL, Dunham HW: Mental Disorders in Urban Areas. New York, Hafner, 1960

Friedman CTH, Faguet RA: Extraordinary Disorders of Human Behavior. New York, Plenum, 1982

German A, Arya OP: Psychiatric morbidity amongst a Uganda student population. Br J Psychiatry 115:1323–1329, 1969

Hemsi LK: Psychiatric morbidity of West Indian immigrants. Soc Psychiatry 2:95–100, 1967

Hes JP: Hypochondriasis in Oriental Jewish immigrants: a preliminary report. Int J Soc Psychiatry 4:18–23, 1958

Hitch PJ, Rock PH: Mental illness among Polish and Russian refugees in Bradford. Br J Psychiatry 137:206–211, 1980

Horowitz MJ: Stress-response syndromes: a review of posttraumatic and adjustment disorders. Hosp Community Psychiatry 37:241–249, 1986

Hull D: Migration, adaptation and illness: a review. Soc Sci Med 13A:25–36, 1979

Kendler KS: Demography of paranoid psychosis (delusional disorder): a review and comparison with schizophrenia and affective illness. Arch Gen Psychiatry 38:890–902, 1982

Kimura SP, Mikolashek PL, Kirk SA: Madness in paradise: psychiatric crises among newcomers in Honolulu. Hawaii Med J 34:275–278, 1975

King H, Locke FB: Health effects of migration: U.S. Chinese in and out of Chinatown. International Migration Review 21:555–576, 1987

Kino FF: Aliens' paranoid reaction. Journal of Mental Science 197:589–594, 1951

Koranyi EK, Kerenzi AB, Sarwer-Foner GJ: Adaptive difficulties of some Hungarian immigrants, IV: the process of adaptation and acculturation. Compr Psychiatry 4:47–57, 1963

Krupinski J: Sociological aspects of mental ill-health in migrants. Soc Sci Med 1:267–281, 1967

Krupinski J, Stoller A, Wallace L: Psychiatric disorders in East European refugees now in Australia. Soc Sci Med 7:31–49, 1973

Lazarus J, Locke BZ, Thomas DS: Migration differentials in mental disease. Milbank Memorial Fund Quarterly 41:25–42, 1963

Lin EMB, Carter WB, Kleinman AM: An exploration of somatization among Asian refugees and immigrants in primary care. Am J Public Health 75:1080–1084, 1985

Lin KM, Masuda M, Tazuma L: Adaptational problems of Vietnamese refugees, III: case studies in clinic and field—adaptive and maladaptive. Psychiatr J Univ Ottawa 7:173–183, 1982

Malzberg B: Mental disorders among native and foreign-born whites in New York State. Am J Psychiatry 93:9–137, 1936

Malzberg B: Migration and mental disease among the white population of New York State, 1949–1951. Hum Biol 34:89–98, 1962

Malzberg B: Mental disease among Irish-born and native whites of Irish parentage in New York State, 1949–51. Mental Hygiene 47:12–42, 1963

Malzberg B: Mental disease among native and foreign-born whites in New York State, 1949–51. Mental Hygiene 48:478–499, 1964

Meszaros AF: Types of displacement reactions among the post revolution Hungarian immigrants. Canadian Psychiatric Association Journal 6:9–19, 1961

Mezey AG: Psychiatric illness in Hungarian refugees. Journal of Mental Science 106:628–637, 1960a

Mezey AG: Personal background, emigration and mental disorder in Hungarian refugees. Journal of Mental Science 106:618–627, 1960b

Morgan MC, Wingard DL, Felice ME: Subcultural differences in alcohol use among youth. Soc Adolescent Medicine 5:191–195, 1984

Nguyen SD: The psychological adjustment and the mental health needs of Southeast Asian refugees. Psychiatric Journal of the University of Ottawa 7:26–35, 1982

Odegaard O: Emigration and insanity: a study of mental disease among the Norwegian born population of Minnesota. Acta Psychiatrica et Neurologica Scandinavica Supplement IV, 1932, pp 1–206

Ostwald P, Bittner E: Life adjustment after severe persecution. Am J Psychiatry 124:1393–1400, 1968

Page JB, Rio L, Sweeney J, et al: Alcohol and adaptation in Miami's Cuban population, in The American Experience With Alcohol: Contrasting Cultural Perspectives. Edited by Bennett LA, Ames GM. New York, Plenum, 1985, pp 315–332

Pasquarelli G: The general medical and associated problems of the Italian-migrant family. Med J Aust 1:65–70, 1966

Pedersen S: Psychopathological reactions to extreme social displacements (refugee neurosis). Psychoanal Rev 36:344–354, 1949

Prange AJ: An interpretation of cultural isolation and aliens' paranoid reaction. Int J Soc Psychiatry 4:254–263, 1959

Roberts BH, Myers JK: Religion, natural origin, immigration, and mental illness. Am J Psychiatry 110:759–764, 1954

Rosen G: Nostalgia: a "forgotten" psychological disorder. Psychol Med 5:340–354, 1975

Ruiz P: Cuban Americans, in Cross-Cultural Psychiatry. Edited by Gaw A. Boston, Wright, 1982, pp 75–86

Salmon TW: The relation of immigration to the prevalence of insanity. American Journal of Insanity 64:53–71, 1907

Seguin CA: Migration and psychosomatic disadaptation. Psychosom Med 18:404–409, 1956

Streltzer J: Psychiatric emergencies in travelers to Hawaii. Compr Psychiatry 20:463–468, 1979

Tans EJ: Cuban unaccompanied minors program: the Wisconsin experience. Child Welfare 61:269–279, 1983

Tseng WS: A paranoid family in Taiwan: a dynamic study of *folie à famille.* Arch Gen Psychiatry 21:55–65, 1969

Tyhurst L: Displacement and migration: a study in social psychiatry. Am J Psychiatry 107:561–568, 1951

Tyhurst L: Displacement and migration: a study in social psychiatry. Am J Psychiatry 107:561–568, 1954

Westermeyer J: Amok, in Extraordinary Disorders of Human Behavior. Edited by Friedman CTH, Faguet R. New York, Plenum, 1982a, pp 173–190

Westermeyer J: Betel nut chewing (letter). JAMA 148:1831–1832, 1982b

Westermeyer J: DSM III psychiatric disorders among Hmong refugees in the United States: a point prevalence study. Am J Psychiatry 145:197–202, 1988

Westermeyer J: National and international strategies to control drug abuse: economic, social and political issues. Adv Alcohol Subst Abuse 8:1–32, 1989

Williams C, Westermeyer J: Psychiatric problems among adolescent Southeast Asian refugees: a descriptive study. J Nerv Ment Dis 171:79–85, 1983

Chapter 4
Clinical Assessment

Chapter 4

Clinical Assessment

Clinical assessment involves several goals. First, adequate psychopathological data must be obtained in order to make a diagnosis. Second, historical information is necessary to reconstruct retrospectively the probable contributors to the patient's condition. While this attempt at ascertaining precipitants to the migrant's current condition may not prove therapeutically beneficial in resolving the current disorder, it may be important in preventing future relapses. Third, data on the patient's strengths and resources form the basis for effective therapeutic inventions. This latter task is especially important for migrants, in whom the usual family and social resources may be absent or altered.

Special approaches to clinical assessment vary with the type of migrant. For example, translation services are needed for many migrants whose primary language is not familiar to the psychiatrist; but such services are not required for migrants from English-speaking countries, returning migrants, and most in-country migrants. Thorough interviewing regarding traumatic experiences is critical in the routine clinical evaluation for many combat veterans and refugees, whereas a few screening questions regarding past trauma suffices for most college students and military inductees.

The psychiatrist's attitudes and approach to assessing the migrant patient are crucial. The assessment task involves suspending judgments, avoiding coming to premature closure, accepting other unfamiliar life-styles, allowing adequate time for rapport to develop, and working through new countertransference issues. New knowledge on language or cultural background may be needed. Team work with an interpreter and others is often required. Assessments are typically complex and require extra time, effort, and creativity. It is important to be patient, accepting, and kind during this process.

Clinical Methods

Establishing optimal rapport often requires extra time and attention. Migrants' mistrust and suspiciousness must be allayed before valid data can be forthcoming on interview. Even returning guest workers, students, and world travelers may believe that the clinician cannot understand them due to their travel-modified norms and values. Migrants who have experienced prejudice in the United States, whether on racial, economic, political, or social grounds, may project negative feelings on any representative of a local social institution, including the psychiatrist. The high incidence of paranoia in many migrants may complicate establishing rapport. Discussion of issues regarding confidentiality and anonymity, as well as legal and ethical practices in the United States, can be beneficial at times.

Despite these various obstacles, excellent rapport can usually be established by observing a few simple steps. First, adequate time should be set aside, so that the patient (and sometimes the family also) can explain the current problem as he, she, or they perceive it. Especially if a translator is used, 1 hour is a minimum, but 1-1/2 or 2 hours is better for the first session. Even 3 hours may be needed if two or more people are interviewed, or if a complicated crisis has arisen (not infrequent among migrants). Second, demonstrating a strong interest in understanding the patient's point of view can be reassuring, especially since the migrant patient may initially believe that no one locally can understand the situation. Third, flexibility and creativity toward the assessment process can be valuable. This flexibility requires a thorough understanding of the goals and methods of assessment, rather than a rigid or "cookbook" approach. And last but not least, the clinician must have good clinical skills and competence in assessing patients of his or her own community, since the task does not become any easier or simpler in assessing migrants (Shuval et al. 1967; Westermeyer 1987a, 1987b).

Interviewing techniques remain much as they are with other patients, with certain modifications. One additional task involves learning about the patient's life in the former residence and the reasons for the migration. This requires extra emphasis on two particular interviewing techniques: (1) facilitating: enabling the patient to express symptoms, thoughts, concerns, feelings, memories, fantasies, and future plans; and (2) clarifying: use of questions and restatements aimed at ensuring that the clinician understands the patient.

Migrant patients, unsure of the psychiatric context or mistrustful of the situation, may begin by reporting numerous somatic symptoms, speaking in brief phrases, complaining about the clinic location or parking, expressing doubt at obtaining any benefit, or weeping for a few minutes. Open-ended questions about physiological functions, such as sleep pattern, appetite, weight change, energy level, and strength often help to get the interview going. Once a dialogue has been established, topics can center on worries, irritability, fears, crying spells, trouble with memory and concentration, suspiciousness, and other psychological symptoms. If the patient insists on remaining with somatic symptoms for a time, a historical review of systems can be introduced earlier than might otherwise be the case. Once rapport has been established, more personal topics such as dreams, anhedonia, and work productivity can be broached. Finally, personal, family, or social problems can be addressed, although some victimized, isolated, or paranoid migrants may not reveal their greatest concerns for weeks or months.

As the interview proceeds, the clinician's own sense of being able to comprehend the story is a critical indicator. Apparent contradictions in the story, emotional reactions that seem excessive, or behaviors that seem inappropriate from the clinician's perspective are possible signs of a misunderstanding on the part of the patient. The patient should also be prompted to ask questions of the psychiatrist when questions or statements are unclear, or when the rationales for certain approaches or procedures are not understood. While at times the interview may take on the characteristics of ethnographic fieldwork or classroom education, the purpose lies entirely in the furtherance of mutual understanding for accurate diagnosis and assessment (Goodenough 1980; Westermeyer 1987a).

Observation of the patient's appearance and behavior is also subject to sociocultural influences. Ethnicity can affect the physical manifestations of stress and psychiatric disorder. For example, Lieblich et al. (1973) demonstrated differences in skin conductance and pulse rate of normal subjects across races and ethnicities. Using an electromyograph on the frontalis muscle, Uchigama et al. (1981) documented lower tension levels in Japanese as compared to Western subjects. British, Mexican, and United States college students distinguished photographs of normal from schizophrenic women better when both rater and subject belonged to the same country (Winkelmayer et al. 1978). Grooming and dress can mislead the examiner unfamiliar with the patient's culture.

A 32-year-old Vietnamese refugee, a former officer and survivor of several years in a concentration camp, was referred by a resettlement agency because of his inability to hold a job. Dress at the interview consisted of a long red robe decorated generously with yellow symbols of Christianity, Buddhism, and several other religions. He responded to questions in a philosophical fashion, weaving religious themes into his responses in a way that led to sermons on subjects that were vaguely related to the original question. An American nurse, a social worker, and a psychiatric resident thought him to be essentially normal, with perhaps slight anxiety. The patient's three Vietnamese roommates, veterans about his same age, expressed alarm at what they considered to be his bizarre costume and idiosyncratic religious ideas. Further interviewing revealed that the patient viewed himself as the reincarnation of Buddha, Christ, and Muhammed. He frequently heard God talking to him, ordering him to save the world. History of his imprisonment in Vietnam revealed that he had been unconscious for several hours following a severe beating about his head with rifle butts. Special tests demonstrated an old skull fracture on X-ray, EEG abnormalities, and an organic pattern of impairment on psychological testing.

Patients' physical placement and activity during the interview, i.e., nonverbal communication along with facial expression and gesticulation, also reflect cultural factors. Anthropologist Hall, in *The Silent Language* (1959), explicated the diverse means by which people of different cultures communicate with one another nonverbally (a field termed *kinesics*) and use space (a field called *proxemics*). His and subsequent studies have demonstrated great similarities among normal subjects in any given culture, but considerable variations among the larger culture regions of the world. Kinesic and proxemic behaviors of American psychiatric patients have shown differences from American normal subjects, but there are obvious dangers in transferring American norms to other cultures. For example, while direct eye contact can signify honesty and openness in Euroamerican culture, the same eye contact can indicate anger or disrespect in other ethnic groups.

Early in work with migrants, it is probably best to ignore one's initial clinical instincts regarding the patient's gesticulation, expression of affect, dress, and mannerisms, and to rely instead on other sources of information. With experience in assessing numerous migrants, the clinician's instincts should again provide a valuable guide in directing the assessment.

History taking in migrants, as observed often in clinical records, commonly begins when the patient arrived in, or returned to the United States. This is understandable to an extent, since the symptoms usually accompany relocation. However, a full understanding of the patient and the clinical picture demands an understanding of the patient's birth, infancy, childhood, adolescence, education, training, skills, size and composition of home community, former life successes and failures, previous migrations, special roles and accomplishments, avocations, and hobbies. With respect to the migration, the clinician should ascertain:

- Premigration status: social network, social and psychological function, premigratory life events;
- Premigration planning: reasons for migrating, duration and extent of planning, goals to be realized;
- Migration experience: duration, difficulty, dangers;
- Resettlement phase vis-à-vis previous life and expectations: roles and activities abandoned, new role and activities adopted, extent of life change.

Clinicians sometimes fail to document premigration histories for specific reasons. These include the belief that they would not understand the relevance of previous life data, the belief that the former life is not relevant to current problems, the belief that the current problem is wholly due to refugee flight and trauma, and the opinion that this information has no prognostic or therapeutic import.

Victimized migrant patients often neglect to mention particular topics of importance unless specifically asked about them. This is especially true for returning combat veterans, prisoners of war, concentration camp survivors, hostages, refugees, and other victims. The reasons for not spontaneously reporting these events are numerous: guilt, shame, wanting to forget, emotional distress in recalling and discussing the events, fear of reprisal, and lack of awareness that these events may be related to the current clinical problem. It therefore falls to the psychiatrist to inquire specifically about certain problematic events and symptoms (e.g., nightmares, intrusive thoughts, remorse).

If the patient comes from an unfamiliar ethnic group, culture, or country, the clinician should obtain some background information on the history, geography, politics, and culture of the area. These general background data should not lead to stereotyping, but rather should be used as a means of putting the patient's personal history into a context.

The Mental Status Examination and its interpretation depend heavily on knowledge of (1) the patient's early ensocialization, (2) the culture of origin, (3) the patient's educational level and literacy, and (4) the duration and extent of the patient's acculturation in the United States (Westermeyer 1985, 1987a). Examples of effects on orientation alone include the following:

- Month, date and year: numerous calendars exist around the world (e.g., Gregorian, Buddhist, Islamic), with scores of different "new year" dates and counting systems;
- Seasons: they vary with distance from the equator, altitude above sea level, and local climatic conditions (such as monsoon);
- Time of day: people with clocks and watches use hours of the day; those without them rely on sun time (e.g., morning, noontime, afternoon, evening, nighttime);
- Floor of the building: many people, such as the French and former French colonies, refer to the first floor as the ground floor or entry floor and the second floor as the first floor.

Evaluation of the patient's cognition depends heavily on the clinician's awareness of the patient's early ensocialization and the patient's acculturation or reentry experiences in the United States. All aspects of intellectual function (e.g., memory, problem solving, perception) can be assessed, but this must be accomplished in a culturally sensitive fashion. Cultural differences among people are particularly related to disparities in their funds of information. Well-educated persons from any background tend to be easier to evaluate (since they ordinarily share the greatest fund of knowledge with the clinician) and illiterate persons are often the more difficult (since most American psychiatrists have little experience with illiterate persons of normal intelligence). For example, well-educated patients usually are oriented for time and place whereas illiterate patients without organic brain damage may have gaps in their orientation to current time and place, have little awareness of national or international events, and not know their birth date (since these comprise irrelevant information in many simple societies).

Proverbs, often used for rapid assessment of intellectual function, can be useful. However, it is generally best to use proverbs to which the patient was exposed during childhood. Those who migrate during adolescence or adulthood are rarely familiar with the proverbs in the new society. It may be possible to figure out the approximate symbolic interpretation but the appreciation of the actual meaning usually requires childhood ensocialization. The reader is invited to match the following Oriental and Occidental proverbs[1]:

Oriental Proverbs

A. There are no waves if there is no wind.
B. If one plants melons one harvests melons.
C. Riding the tiger.
D. The wood has already been burned.
E. One hair from nine oxen.
F. Paper cannot wrap fire.

Occidental Proverbs

1. A drop in the bucket.
2. Biting off more than you can chew.
3. Where there's smoke there's fire.
4. It's water over the dam.
5. The truth will out.
6. As ye sow so shall ye reap.

Education and life experience can greatly affect assessment of intelligence. Those migrants of normal intelligence who have not attended school can usually add single numbers but not double numbers. Illiterate individuals who have worked as merchants or taxi drivers in societies with currency can usually subtract, although their fellow illiterate farmers and laborers often cannot do so. Their current fund of knowledge depends greatly on the time since emigration, literacy, and progress of acculturation. Refugees and other victimized for-

[1]Key: A=3; B=6; C=2; D=4; E=1; F=5

eigners may perceive "fund of information" questions as being political in nature, and either feign ignorance or refuse to answer. Ability to recognize and name certain objects (e.g., coins, pen, or pencil) is dependent on being familiar with them. Immediate, recent, intermediate, and remote memory tasks need not differ so greatly across cultures. Nonetheless, the clinician must appreciate that which is worth remembering from the patient's standpoint—and not the clinician's standpoint. For example, people in some groups eat the same breakfast or dinner every day, so that question does not distinguish intermediate memory well. Former addresses can be long remembered by those who relocate once or twice in a lifetime, but not by those who relocate every year or two. Analysis of the patient's problem-solving abilities can present challenges to the clinician unfamiliar with the range of problems and alternative resolutions in the patient's culture.

Paper-and-pencil tests that do not require linguistic skills (such as the Bender Gestalt test) can be quite useful across cultures and languages, if the patient has had experience with paper and pencil. Otherwise, such tests can be grossly misleading. Illiterate persons who have learned to sign their names to documents, such as applications, contracts, and checks, may not be able to write anything else.

Directions to undertake certain tasks can be biased if terms or concepts are unfamiliar to the patient or cannot be translated into the patient's language. An example is the word *lap* in the common assessment request, "Put this object in your lap." This concept and the term for it are absent in some societies that traditionally did not have chairs. One would thus have to say to a sitting person, "Put this object on your upper legs" or some similar translation.

Several cross-cultural and cross-language studies have been conducted on the Mini-Mental Status Examination (MMSE), using translations of this instrument. These data indicate that translations are reasonably valid with subjects less than age 65 years having more than eight grades of education. Even when the items are sensitive to cultural differences, the rate of false-positive MMSEs in poorly educated or elderly subjects is unacceptably high (Escobar et al. 1986).

Evaluation of mood and affect may be as straightforward as with nonmigrant patients, or quite complex. The greater the cultural "gap" between patient and clinician, and the more unfamiliar the clinician is with the patient's culture, the more potential error there is in recognizing emotional anguish. "Smiling" depression, seen more often in the United States a few decades ago but now relatively rare, occurs regularly in some migrant groups that value containment of negative emotions. This masklike smile can accompany severe melancholic and even psychotic depressions.

Collateral sources of data are often key elements in the evaluation and diagnosis of migrants. Records from previous treatment facilities, information from friends and family, and cultural data on behavioral norms can be important. Ethnographic, historical, and social psychological data from books, periodicals, journals, or social scientists can prove useful in placing the clinical data into a social, cultural, and historical context. The patient, the family, and the interpreter may all contribute to understanding the patient and the clinical problem.

One of these sources of help is the consultant with special migration-related expertise. This person may be a highly trained anthropologist, a military historian, an attorney familiar with immigration law, a staff member from the Immigration and Naturalization Service (INS), or other person with special knowledge. Expatriate peers or fellow migrants can provide background information that can aid in distinguishing expected from unusual behavior, religious beliefs from fixed delusions, or culturally consistent expressions from meaningless phrases.

Communication: Language, Translation, and Interpretation

Some migrant patients do not have adequate skills in English to serve the purposes of history taking. Translation services are therefore required. This raises several special problems for psychiatric assessment, since we are highly reliant on verbal and nonverbal communication for obtaining a thorough history and performing a Mental Status Examination. Language differences pose a barrier that can be transcended, however.

Selecting a language for psychiatric assessment can be a complex process. Migrant patients frequently speak more than one language, including perhaps the clinician's language. Consequently it may seem logical to conduct the interview in the language common to the patient and clinician, without the services of an interpreter. This may not be the best strategy if the language was acquired in a classroom setting and never spoken in an intimate face-to-face living situation. Symptom expression may be altered in a second language. Speakers may be able to communicate their thoughts adequately in a language used in a school, work, or market setting, but they may be unable to communicate their feelings freely. This is not unusual when one considers that emotionally colored expression and unguarded dialogue occur among close family members, friends, and relatives. The extra effort speaking in a second language can result in an inordinately abbreviated history, bereft of the emotional content so critical to psychiatric interviewing. Those experiencing severe anxiety, despair, or cognitive slippage can even be less adept than usual in speaking their second language. Various clinical misadventures, including suicides that were potentially preventable, have ensued when the clinician has not had a true picture of a patient's actual condition due to linguistic obstacles (DelCastillo 1970; Edgerton and Karno 1971; Peck 1974; Sabin 1975).

Alternatively, the clinician may be tempted to interview a patient using a second language studied in school or used on vacation trips. Unless the clinician has lived and worked in the language, the denotative and connotative dimensions of the language may not be appreciated even by a competent clinician.

Occasionally the patient may not want an interpreter, even though the clinician may perceive a need for one. Refusal itself can be a useful datum. Patients may be fearful that a fellow national might know certain things about them, or may feel insulted about their language skills, or may want to impress the psychiatrist with their "good English." It can be useful to have the interpreter in the room even while the patient is responding mostly in English in order to provide help with certain of the clinician's questions (which may not be comprehensible to the patient) or with particular words or phrases which the patient does not know in English.

Skill in working with an interpreter is critical for the clinician seeing a variety of migrant patients. Ability to work with various interpreters, patients, and languages requires experience. Ideally, the clinician new to this task should observe experienced clinicians working with different interpreters, in order to adopt congenial styles and methods. Supervision of clinical work with interpreters is also valuable, if the supervisor has had experience. In order to appreciate the demands on the interpreter, the psychiatrist accomplished in two languages might try to translate between a patient and a colleague or nurse. These latter experiences can orient the clinician to the many nuances and demands that interpretation involves, as well as helping the clinician to empathize with interpreters and to understand interpreting process. The psychiatrist must learn to ask translatable questions and to educate, confront, and interpret in translatable terms and statements (Marcos 1979; Marcos et al. 1973; Westermeyer 1987b).

Miscommunication can ensue if the clinical interpreter is not trained for and skilled in psychiatric interviewing. One of these skills involves translation or the ability to exchange words from one language for those of another language while retaining the same meaning. The term *translation* usually refers to written work, which is judged by its denotative accuracy. It requires good command of two languages, usually requiring several years of study in the language. A more subtle skill is *interpretation,* which refers to transmission of connotative as well as denotative meaning; it usually applies to dialogue rather than to written materials. Interpretation requires

74

that the interpreter understand the task at hand, its purpose, and the means for achieving it. For example, a medical interpreter would be trained in medical terminology, know about various aspects of the doctor-patient relationship (e.g., confidentiality), and be familiar with and comfortable in the clinical setting. Psychiatric interpreters likewise should be familiar with elements of psychiatric interviewing and certain clinical concepts and methods, such as the following: medical, psychiatric, psychological, and social terminology; technique of psychiatric interviewing (e.g., closed-and open-ended questions, facilitation, clarification, confrontation); normal and abnormal psychology, anatomy, physiology; types of psychotherapies, sociotherapies, and somatotherapies; the importance of verbal as well as nonverbal communication in psychiatric interviewing; cultural influences on Mental Status Examination; and methods of asking about matters that do not come up in ordinary conversation, such as inquiring about hallucinations, delusions, suicidal plans and impulses, paranoid symptoms, sexual problems, financial matters, family conflicts, and other information apt to be considered personal.

The goal of diagnostic interviewing is to enable patients who are experiencing a given symptom to endorse questions regarding the symptoms (or not endorse them, if the symptom is asked). Auditory hallucinations are an example. In some languages, a literal translation of the question "Do you hear voices?" may be endorsed by virtually everyone. The following are examples of literal translations apt to elicit valid responses for auditory hallucinations (depending on the language) are as follows:"Do you hear voices when no one else hears them?"; "Do you hear noises that sound like people speaking?"; or "Do you hear people speaking even though no one is present?".

Models of translation services currently being employed broadly fall into three different types. One can be referred to as the triangle model shown in Figure 1. Six types of communications or relationships can be envisioned, as compared to the simpler two-way model in Figure 2 (i.e., transference and countertransference) that exists when a patient and psychiatrist work together. While the triangle model reflects the actual situation most accurately and brings the skills of the psychiatrist most directly to the patient, it also places the greatest demands on the psychiatrist in terms of keeping all six communication-relationship channels in mind. With time and experience, this task lightens appreciably. The breaks in verbal communications, which occur while the interpreter is speaking to the patient, permit the psychiatrist to observe both the patient and the translator, to attend to their nonverbal behavior, and to frame the next question in a fashion that can be effectively and efficiently translated. This author prefers to have the three parties seated in an equilateral triangle as depicted in Figure 1, so that each member can see the other two. Other clinicians prefer the interpreter to the side (giving prominence to the psychiatrist) or the psychiatrist to the side (giving prominence to the psychiatric interpreter). The triangle model does help raise to a conscious level the transference-countertransfer-

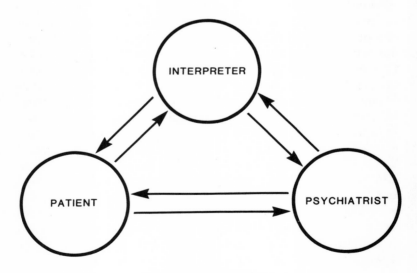

Figure 1. Triangle Model

ence between the patient and interpreter (which are important factors in the assessment, and even more so in the treatment), as well as the mutual working relationship between the psychiatrist and the psychiatric interpreter, and the transference-countertransference between the patient and the psychiatrist. It lends weight to the fact that the psychiatrist and the psychiatric interpreter have a mutual relationship, that each must trust the other, and that they must understand one another's tasks and appreciate one another's skills. The quality between the three roles in Figure 1 should not be equated with professional, legal, or symbolic status. While the voluntary patient can "hire or fire" the other two, there can be the imposing physical fact of two staff against one patient. Alternately, the easily threatened clinician, faced by two persons of the same language and usually same culture or race, may feel overwhelmed. The psychiatrist is in fact, legally and ethically, in charge of the interpreter and the interview process—a fact that must be appreciated by the interpreter.

The two-way model can be referred to as "the black box approach," depicted in Figure 2. This model treats the interpreter as a word unscrambler, who merely takes messages from one person and passes them on to the other, without interposing between the patient and the clinician. This model reflects how many psychiatrists and interpreters, new to this clinical task, perceive their mutual roles. It is a model that is indeed sought after in many settings, such as multilingual conferences and international meetings. Eventually, both psychiatrists and interpreters become disenchanted with this model. Psychia-

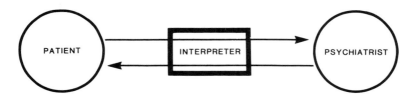

Figure 2. "Black Box" or Two-Way Model

trists become increasingly aware that the interpreter is not, and cannot be a "black box" in the psychiatric interview. Interpreters relegated to this role similarly find it impossible, and demeaning as well (since their actual role is more complex and demanding). Most psychiatrists starting with this model move to the "triangle model" described earlier. Others move to a third model described next.

In this model the psychiatrist abandons all attempts to deal with the complexities of translation and interpretation, assigning the bilingual worker to a status of a "junior clinician." As depicted in Figure 3, the bilingual worker sees the patient alone and then reports back to the psychiatrist in charge of the case at another time and place. The psychiatrist then supervises the bilingual worker, but does not see the patient. If the bilingual worker has appropriate clinical education, training, certification, and licensure, this junior clinician model of course is as valid as supervising a professional who happens not to be bilingual. If the bilingual worker is not professionally trained, this model possesses certain obvious legal and ethical considerations when used exclusively. (Later during therapy,

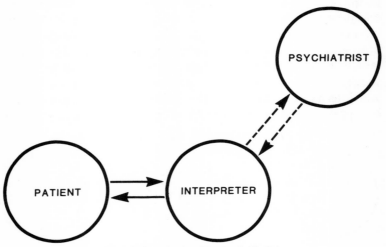

Figure 3. "Junior Clinician" Model

psychiatrists relying primarily on the "triangle model" may also employ this "junior clinician" model intermittently, depending on the experience, skill, and training of the bilingual worker, while still continuing to see the patient with the worker on a regular basis.)

Emergency translators, although clearly a second choice, must be used from time to time. Absence of a bilingual worker on the staff, medical emergencies, crises after hours or on the weekend, and innumerable other situations give rise to the necessity to work with whomever is at hand. Such persons include relatives, friends, housekeeping or janitorial staff at the hospital, foreign students in the community, or even other patients. Appreciation of the complexities and expertise needed for certain questions and topics enables the clinician to guide the interview toward obtaining reliable information, while skirting topics likely to lead to false information (which is always worse than no information). Even the most unsophisticated translator can usually help with the following: open-ended questions (i.e., facilitation), obtaining demographic data, and questions regarding physical and physiological symptoms. Depending on the patient, the emergency translator, and the context, it may be possible to ask directed questions about certain psychological symptoms, such as worry, irritability, sleep disturbances, anxiety symptoms, phobias, memory, concentration, mood changes, and behavioral changes. Generally it is not feasible to pursue such topics as suicide, hallucinations, delusions, sexual dysfunction, family problems, or a detailed social history. It frequently occurs that fellow expatriates attempt to "normalize" the patient's psychopathology by not translating material relevant to suicide, paranoid ideation, or other topics that embarrass the translator or cause the translator to "protect" the patient from "medical authorities"—not an extraordinary event if one remembers the mistrust and suspiciousness manifest in many migrants who are otherwise functional in society.

Most translation and interpretation takes place in a sequential fashion, with only one person speaking at a time.

That is, the interpreter listens to the patient or to the psychiatrist and then speaks. This process takes at least twice as much time, adding appreciably to the cost of assessment and treatment. Concurrent interpretation consists of the interpreter translating and speaking while the patient or psychiatrist is speaking. This latter method has been adopted from the process employed at multilingual conferences and international meetings and is being used in some areas of New York City for English-Spanish translation. Although concurrent interpretation saves time, it can have several disadvantages: i.e., greater stress on and more rapid fatigue of the interpreter; more possibilities for error; greater emphasis on denotative translation at the expense of connotative interpretation; more effort and stress on the psychiatrist who has to simultaneously scan the patient, the translator, and himself or herself while the interview is proceeding at twice the rate of the sequential interview. Concurrent translators do not usually perform other clinical responsibilities (e.g., education, support, crisis intervention, outreach), and they tend to fit into the "black box" model of interpretation.

Forensic evaluation in the psychiatric setting can add further to the complexity, time, and expense of interpretation. It is not unusual to have two, or even three interpreters present at the assessment. These might include the regular psychiatric interpreter or bilingual staff worker, an interpreter for the prosecution or plaintiff, and an interpreter for the defendant. Many approaches can be used to manage this type of interview, but a standard approach is to complete the assessment (or subsections of it) with the regular psychiatric interpreter and then to ask if there are disagreements regarding interpretations that should be clarified. The legal interpreters must understand that the clinic is not a court of law, and their attendance at the interview is to ensure that all sides concur on the accuracy and meaning of the translation. Legal interpreters are acquainted with the courtroom context in which only two or three facts may be covered in an hour, with much attention directed to the validity of these facts. In an hour of psychiatric interviewing, several hundred data bits (process as well as content) may be forthcoming, with much attention paid to internal reliability of interview data, but little paid to external validity.

Related to translation and interpretation is the matter of American dialects in the English language. Differences exist in terms, idiom, connotation, accent, grammar, and linguistic style. These may vary by region, age, sex, race, and ethnicity. Although interpreters are not involved if both patient and clinician are native English speakers, nonetheless the clinician should be sensitive to language issues if a notable dialectical difference exists. Clarification helps immeasurably early on, and with time most clinicians can adapt to their patients' dialects.

Bilingual Psychiatric Assistant

In clinical facilities treating many migrants speaking a foreign language, the psychiatric interpreter is often a member of the psychiatric team. Other responsibilities shouldered by the psychiatric interpreter may include orientation to the assessment process, education of the family regarding a patient's psychopathology, or discussion of psychiatric treatment. Those with professional training in health or social services may assume additional responsibilities with supervision, such as crisis intervention, brief supportive or directive counseling, and outreach. When functioning as a team member, the psychiatric interpreter is often referred to as a bilingual psychiatric assistant. Psychiatrists, other physicians, psychologists, social workers, and nurses may have a professional identity and also be able to interpret for other team members (Kline et al. 1980; Sabin 1975).

Bilingual psychiatric workers are often employed for work with refugees, since this group of migrants relocates in large numbers and has high rates of psychiatric disorder. It requires 1 or 2 years of course work and on-the-job training for these workers to become efficient and competent at their work. Those who remain with this work are mostly in their twenties upon arrival in the United States and have some background in the medical field, social services, or teaching. Salaries must be competitive to attract and keep high-quality people to this difficult work. Compensated school time can help in attracting upwardly mobile persons who are going on for professional degrees and certification.

Since these workers have often been through the same losses and traumas as their patients, the work can be stressful for them. Members of the local refugee community call upon them at home as well as at work. As people operating at the boundary of the majority society and the refugee community, they are naturally at risk to feelings of marginality.

Among 10 refugee bilingual psychiatric workers employed in one refugee program over a several-year period, 8 required psychiatric treatment at some point. Only 1 was briefly hospitalized; the others responded to outpatient care. Four missed no work; the 4 others missed a few days to a few weeks. Two people could not resume work with refugees; the other 6 returned to their jobs. Precipitants included divorce (2 cases), theft from the home (2 cases), assaults (1 by a psychotic patient, 1 a rape), and no known cause (2 cases). Onset varied from 2 to 10 years after arrival in the United States. Most common diagnosis in the 8 bilingual psychiatric workers was major depression ($n = 7$), although pathogenic substance use occurred in 1 of these cases and paranoid features in 2 of these cases. Diagnosis in the remaining person, whose disorder started later while employed in another program, was paranoid psychosis. These refugee workers sought treatment relatively soon after onset of symptoms (i.e., more like typical American patients, rather than delayed as is typical of refugee patients) and outcomes were fair to excellent in 7 of the 8 cases. The paranoid patient did not cooperate with care and still is episodically symptomatic. This small sample suggests that knowledge and experience in the psychiatric field is not necessarily "immunizing" for bilingual psychiatric assistants, but they do use psychiatric services appropriately and with reasonably good outcomes in most cases.

Special Issues in Assessing Migrants

Spiegel (1976) has described the cultural dimensions of transference and countertransference. Patients can experience thoughts and feelings about the clinician by virtue of the latter's apparent race, national origin, or ethnic affiliation. The history of the patient's ethnic group vis-à-vis the psychiatrist's ethnic group can affect this. For example, American Indian people raised from childhood to distrust authority figures in the majority society (based on abundant historical precedent) may have serious difficulty in trusting a non-Indian psychiatrist—and perhaps even an Indian psychiatrist from a tribe that had been a traditional enemy. Transference of this type can result in delay of clinical care and premature departure from treatment (Westermeyer 1987a, 1987b). Countertransference issues resemble transference issues. Psychiatrists whose family or person has been victimized by someone of another group (e.g., in war, or in the United States by rape, assault, robbery) may have feelings that consciously or unconsciously generalize to that entire group, and to the particular patient being assessed. Transference and countertransference can be unrealistically positive, as well as negative. For example, some patients may demean the competence of clinicians belonging to their own ethnic group—a symptom of poor ethnic identity—and ascribe greater abilities to physicians of other ethnic groups. For example, my Irish immigrant relatives in the United States, 40 years ago, sought the services of a non-Irish physician if they believed their malady was life-threatening, although they consulted Irish-American physicians for more prosaic illnesses. Many of these people, involuntary immigrants on politicoeconomic bases around 1900, harbored hostility against their own nation, which had not been able to establish itself, and doubt regarding any Irish competence. This anger and doubt resulted in unrealistically negative expectations toward Irish-American physicians and unrealistically positive expectations toward non-Irish physicians, in the face of anxiety-provoking symptoms.

Likewise, psychiatrists can develop problematic positive countertransference under certain circumstances. For example, the psychiatrist may idealize the strength, resilience, and traditions of certain groups and their members, thereby ascribing false strengths or abilities to the patient. This is apt to occur with returning combat veterans and prisoners of war, concentration camp survivors, refugees, and American Indians (whose history and traditions have been both demeaned and idealized in the mass media). Individual and group supervision of clinical work and seminars on migrant psychiatry are key to recognizing and dealing with these transference-countertransference issues.

Somatization can present special problems to clinicians unfamiliar with this common presentation in migrants. In fact, it usually presents no problem when properly approached. As with nonmigrant patients, the psychiatrist should use the following steps for interviewing the somatizing patient:

1. Facilitate full expression of the patient's somatic symptoms, along with information about social, psychological, and environmental precipitants, factors that ameliorate or exacerbate the symptoms (this step alone provides an entree to psychosocial issues in most migrants);
2. Complete a full review of physiological systems, with particular attention to sleep, appetite, weight, strength, energy, and somatic symptoms of anxiety and depression (e.g., tachycardia, dyspnea, constipation, anorexia);
3. Ask direct questions about psychological symptoms, since these patients rarely volunteer these symptoms but do endorse these symptoms if they are present; these include worry, irritability, gloomy future, crying spells, restlessness, phobias, nightmares, mood changes, difficulties in problem solving, concentration and memory impairment, diurnal vari-

ation in symptoms, mistrust, suspiciousness, ideas of reference, hallucinations, bothersome or intrusive thoughts, suicidal or homicidal impulses or plans;
4. An extensive and detailed social history to identify precipitants, since somatizing patients have often not made the link between the pathogenic factors and their symptoms;
5. Careful mental status and biomedical evaluation to rule out the common biomedical conditions seen in migrants (i.e., endocrine, chronic infectious, nutritive, and organic brain disorders).

Even among nonmigrants in certain countries, somatization often occurs in psychiatric patients as "an idiom of psychosocial distress" (Nichter 1981). Depressive disorders (especially melancholic and psychotic depression) and various anxiety disorders [e.g., posttraumatic stress disorder (PTSD), social phobia, panic attacks] account for the overwhelming majority of somatic presentations in migrants. Somatoform disorder is infrequent: this author identified only 3 cases among 300 refugees and immigrants in a psychiatric clinic. It must be kept in mind that somatization is a symptom, not a disorder. It can occur with any and all Axis I and Axis II psychiatric diagnoses, and at any age. Emotional distress associated with somatic symptoms may not necessarily compose somatization; biomedical disease must also be considered.

Careful psychiatric history along with awareness of special biomedical conditions in migrants can aid the psychiatrist in identifying biomedical illnesses.

A 27-year-old single American woman returning home from Europe experienced severe anxiety symptoms. History revealed several stresses in Europe: disappointment at failure of her artistic aspirations; theft of all her money, traveler's checks, and identification; and grudging response of local authorities, banks, the American embassy, and family at home to assist her in dealing with her losses. Evaluation revealed tachycardia, weight loss despite increased food intake, and tremor. Laboratory tests revealed moderately severe hyperthyroidism. The patient responded to treatment for this condition; no further psychiatric care was needed.

Such patients should be seen at intervals throughout their course of biomedical care in order to assure the resolution of their psychiatric symptoms. Psychiatric care may still be needed for patients whose biomedical conditions cannot be cured or whose psychiatric symptoms persisted despite adequate care of the biomedical problem.

A 36-year-old refugee widow presented with symptoms of major depression, melancholic type, beginning two years previously upon arrival in the United States. However, two of her symptoms—fatigue and amenorrhea—had begun several years ago following the birth of her last child, which had involved a massive hemorrhage. Laboratory tests demonstrated Simmond's disease. Endocrine replacement for her panhypopituitarism failed to alleviate her depressive symptoms, which subsequently responded to psychiatric treatment.

The DSM-III-R diagnosis of posttraumatic stress disorder (PTSD) can be made fairly easily by asking several questions regarding nightmares, intrusive daytime thoughts, disturbing déjà vu experiences, emotional distancing and numbing, and associated anxiety and depressive symptoms. It is also important to ascertain the duration, frequency, severity, and waxing-waning pattern of these symptoms, along with the extent of associated social disability. These patients, unlike those victims of violence who do not have PTSD, seldom volunteer the story of the victimization or violence. Consequently, the psychiatrist must ask directed questions about violent experiences before, during, and after the migration experience. Since this type of interviewing can be stressful, and can even produce a period of clinical deterioration, it is best left to the post-assessment period, when a treatment plan has been recommended to the patient, accepted, and instituted. (PTSD interviewing is an example of that vague interface between assessment and treatment, since more extensive assessment should only be undertaken in a context of treatment.)

Paranoid symptoms, common in many migrants, also present problems in assessment. Patients rarely volunteer these anger-associated symptoms and may actually hide them if they involve fantasies of assault, revenge, or homicide. It therefore falls to the psychiatrist to aid the patient in expressing these symptoms and in ensuring that loss of self-esteem or "face" does not ensue. The following general principles of psychiatric interviewing apply to assessment:

• Begin with routine questions that are least threatening (e.g., "Do you have trouble trusting people since you returned to the U.S.?" or "Are you suspicious of people now even when you have no reason to be so?");
• Progress to more flagrant symptoms only if milder symptoms are endorsed (e.g., "If you see two people talking, but cannot hear them, is there a tendency to think that they are talking about you?" and "Do you ever hear voices threatening you?" and "Do you sometimes feel that there is a plot against you?").

As with somatization, paranoid symptoms attend a wide variety of symptoms among refugees. These include affective disorders, chronic adjustment syndromes, social phobias, PTSD, and organic brain syndromes. Paranoid conditions include paranoid personality, brief paranoid reactions, longer lasting paranoid psychosis, shared delusional disorder, and paranoid schizophrenia. Establishing the presence of paranoid symptoms is only the first step in ascertaining the disorder with which they are associated.

Delusions are not always readily distinguished from cultural beliefs in assessing patients who express ideas unfamiliar to the psychiatrist (Westermeyer 1988). Familiarity with the patient's culture, their world views and traditional beliefs, can greatly ease the task; but no one can be familiar with all cultures. Collateral information from a few people who are familiar with or are members of the patient's culture can usually clarify whether the patient is expressing culture-related beliefs (e.g., in some societies, speaking with ghosts of the deceased during dreams) or delusions. The structure of the idea can also be a tip-off, since delusions around the world fall into a relatively small number of categories (e.g., nihilistic, somatic, grandiose, paranoid or persecutory, organic paraphrenic). Even the content of delusions in most cultures is secular and readily recognized as typical themes observed everywhere (e.g., projected hostility, hypochondriacal delusions of fatal disease). Culture-related content of a kind that might confuse the clinician (usually religious) have been observed in a minority of cases from the United States, Middle East, Africa, and Asia (Bazzouli and Al-Issa 1966; Benedict and Jacks 1954; El-Islam and Malasi 1985; El Sendiony 1976; Opler 1959; Weinstein 1962; Westermeyer 1988; Wittkower et al. 1960). Traditional and religious content in delusions (e.g., involving sorcery, spiritual powers) have been observed in association with provincial (i.e., nonmetropolitan) residence, lower social class, less education, more intense religious ensocialization during childhood, and greater support for magical or mythical beliefs in culturally supported institutions (e.g., church, school). Historical studies of delusions in England and Switzerland indicate a decline in traditional or religious content and an increase in secular themes over time (Klaf and Hamilton 1973; Steinbrunner and Scharfetter 1976). In addition to the structure and content of the delusional ideas, associated symptoms and course of the disorder also contribute toward differentiating delusion from belief.

Dreams and nightmares are often reported by patients, especially those with PTSD (Tyhurst 1951). Content and personal significance of dreams and ghosts can cause confusion in diagnosis, due to differences in beliefs and attitudes around the world. Familiarity with traditional views of dreams and ghosts in certain societies along with associated symptoms and behaviors contributes to the assessment.

A personal ethnographic history can be a valuable part of the social history. This may be obtained during interview, or the patient might be assigned to do an autobiography as a part of "homework" assignments between sessions. Topics to be considered include the following:

- Ethnicity of parents and grandparents (i.e., country of origin, religion, language, migrations, traditional roles and skills);
- Early ensocialization experiences of the patient (i.e., language, rituals, size and type of home community, family religious practice);
- Adolescent rites and activities to assume adult status, persistence or abandonment of family ethnicity including behaviors, values, and attitudes;
- Marriage (into same or different ethnic group), establishment of ethnic practices in the new family of marriage;
- Current ethnic practice in terms of ceremonies, rituals, customs, avocations, ethnic affiliations and associations, use of free time and disposable income, contact with relatives, religious practice.

Assessment of the illiterate patient presents special challenges to most United States psychiatrists unfamiliar with illiterate persons except among preschool children and the moderately to severely mentally retarded. Lack of experience with such people can lead the clinician mistakenly to view illiterate persons as childlike (e.g., innocent, immature, inexperienced, unknowledgeable) and/or mentally retarded (i.e., lacking in problem-solving skill and ability to acquire and utilize new information). These mistaken conclusions may be reinforced by the illiterate patient's inability to perform numerous tasks learned early in school (e.g., reading, writing, complex arithmetic) and lack of knowledge on many topics learned in school or discovered through reading (e.g., elementary facts regarding geography, history, literature, social science, biology, chemistry, physics, government, law, nutrition). Lack of school-based skills and knowledge does not indicate lack of intelligence, maturity, insight, or the ability to collaborate in psychiatric assessment and treatment. Experience with illiterate patients enables the clinician to recognize their individual assets and liabilities, while not giving way to stereotypes formed from other groups of people. Classical clinical methods (such as the Mental Status Examination, paper-and-pencil tasks) can be grossly misleading, so that the psychiatrist is forced to choose indices of skill and attainment relative to the illiterate patient's background (e.g., number and type of special roles or skills, problem-solving abilities, maturity and wisdom in dealing with life's vicissitudes, recent and remote memory of relevant facts, leadership roles and abilities).

The culturally naïve psychiatrist may have more difficulty with cross-cultural diagnosis, at least for certain diagnoses, as compared to psychiatrists who have had more cross-cultural experience. For example, 9 psychiatrists from technically developed countries (trained in their own countries) were compared with 4 psychiatrists from developing countries (trained in developed countries) (Leff 1974). These 13 psychiatrists were presented with videotapes of 26 patients from their respective countries, along with a translation of the interview. All 13 psychiatrists showed good interrater agreement with patients from the developed countries, but only those 4 psychiatrists from the developing countries had high reliabilities on patients from the developing countries. In another study (Westermeyer and Sines 1979), two "Asia-experienced" clinicians were compared against two "Asia-naïve" clinicians, using 35 written case reports of Asians accompanied by a photograph of the subject. (The two "Asia-naïve" clinicians had never been to Asia, although they had considerable experience with other cultures in and out of the United States.) Using the Kappa score (Fleiss 1973) as a measure of interrater reliability, the "Asia-experienced" and "Asia-naïve" raters scored essentially the same for the diagnoses of schizophrenia, affective psychosis, and organic psychosis. However, when the folk syndrome of *baa* (crazy or insane) was compared with the psychiatric diagnosis of psychosis, the "Asia-experienced" clinicians showed higher Kappa scores (i.e., .63 and .68) indicating reasonably good agreement with local villagers, and the "Asia-naïve" clinicians obtained lower Kappa scores (i.e., .21 and .52) indicating poorer agreement with the villagers (Westermeyer and Zimmerman 1981).

The errors of culturally inexperienced clinicians can include overdiagnosis (i.e., diagnosing a nonpsychotic depressed person as psychotic), underdiagnosis (i.e., diagnosing a psychotic person as being nonpsychotic), and misdiagnosis (i.e., diagnosing a depressed person as schizophrenic) (Westermeyer 1987a, 1987b). Taken together, the research reports show that "culturally naïve" clinicians can often make reliable diagnoses, especially for the more severe, stereotypical psychotic disorders; but they are less skilled as contrasted with "culturally experienced" clinicians at distinguishing most psychotic conditions. These diagnostic errors are not merely academic misadventures, but can have serious practical implications.

> A 48-year-old ethnic Chinese woman from Vietnam had been treated for psychotic depression with antipsychotic and antidepressant medication, along with brief monthly outpatient visits. On this regimen, the patient had lost more weight and become less physically active and more hopeless. The psychiatrist's diagnosis of psychosis had been based on the woman's belief that her deceased mother, who had been appearing in her dreams, had traveled from the place of the dead in order to induce the patient's death and accompany her to the next world. Her belief was not delusional, but a culturally consistent dream interpretation. This patient responded well after the antipsychotic medication was discontinued, the antidepressant medication was reduced in dosage (to therapeutic blood levels), and weekly psychotherapy was instituted.

Special Assessment Procedures

The clinical instruments used in assessing nonmigrants apply to migrants, but with certain alterations or special considerations. Translation and restandardization (or "renorming") of self-rating scales and psychometrics pose the main obstacles to using these instruments. Fortunately, extensive experience with translation and restandardization has been acquired over the last few decades (Boleloucky and Horwath 1974; Brislin 1970; Butcher and Garcia 1978; Butcher and Gur 1974; Chien 1978; Kim et al. 1978; Westermeyer 1986; Westermeyer et al. 1983a). Out of these experiences, the following general format for translation and restandardization of rating scales and psychometrics into the new language has evolved:

1. Initial translation should be undertaken by someone with at least several years of living in both cultures and fluency in both languages.
2. The initial translation should then be critiqued and modified by a panel of bilingual persons representing both sexes, a range of ages and classes, diverse educational levels, and various levels of psychological sophistication.
3. Next, the instrument should be back-translated by a fluent bilingual person who has not been involved in the translation process thus far. If possible, a few to several different people (varied by demographic background) should do back translations so as to detect biased or unclear translation. (In one study, the original panel had phrased all statements to fit men, so that women could not respond to certain items. In another, the translation for one item assumed that the subject had to be married, although single persons were expected to complete all items on the instrument.)
4. A small pilot study should next be conducted on several to a dozen persons unfamiliar with the instrument. Spontaneous feedback from their personal experience in being assessed with the instrument is invited. This should complete the first translation phase.
5. Restandardization should then be undertaken in two separate populations. One of these should be a general population of "normal" persons from the target population. The other should be a clinical population manifesting the disorder being assessed by the instrument (e.g., depression, mental retardation, substance abuse).

6. Once data have been collected in these two different groups, the next step consists of item analysis, subscale analysis (if there are subscales), and scale analysis. This process, too technical to describe here, requires special expertise and tools (i.e., computers, statistics).
7. Based on the latter analysis, further modifications or even deletions may be implemented. This can lead to another round of translation and restandardization.

Certain instruments are easier to translate and restandardize than others. Those with largely biological and physiological symptoms and few or no idiomatic expressions are relatively simple; most self-rating scales fall into this category. Language-free tests and subscales do not require any translation but they may need restandardization; examples include draw a person/house/tree/family, tests for organic impairment such as the Bender Gestalt and parts of the Reitan battery, and certain parts of intelligence tests such as the Wechsler Adult Intelligence Scale (WAIS) and the Wechsler Intelligence Scale for Children (WISC). Most difficult to translate and reinterpret are empirical tests for personality and psychopathology, since these tests rely on numerous items with strongly culture-bound items. Despite obstacles, this type of translation and interpretation can be done. For example, Butcher and co-workers around the world have translated and restandardized the Minnesota Multiphasic Personality Inventory (MMPI) into many languages, including not only most European languages and subdialects of Spanish in Latin America, but also into Thai, Japanese, and Chinese (Mandarin) (Butcher and Garcia 1978; Butcher and Gur 1974; Butcher and Pancheri 1976; Butcher and Spielberger 1985). Instruments that have been both inadequately translated and evaluated can have untoward consequences (Berkanovic 1980).

Self-rating scales have been employed for clinical and epidemiological studies of various groups of migrants. These have mostly consisted of instruments translated and restandardized in the migrant's primary language (Cochrane et al. 1977; Kinzie and Manson 1987; Lin et al. 1979; Westermeyer 1986; Westermeyer et al. 1983a). Kinzie and co-workers (1982) have developed a self-rating scale for Vietnamese refugees, using some idiomatic complaints frequent in this group. In addition to their use for research studies, self-rating scales have certain practical applications. They are an inexpensive screening instrument for certain migrants at high risk to psychiatric disorder (e.g., refugees in medical clinics and on welfare rolls). In psychiatric settings, self-rating scales can be used to follow patients over time in order to assess therapeutic response. For children, self-rating scales can be supplemented by parent-rated scales and teacher-rated scales on the children. Among adults, the General Health Questionnaire, Zung Depression Scale, 90-item Symptom Checklist, and Cornell Medical Index have been widely used in cross-cultural and migrant studies (Derogatis et al. 1971, 1973; Zung 1975).

Psychological testing of migrant patients should be in the hands of a competent psychologist trained in cross-cultural/cross-language psychological assessment, and the assessment of migrants. Those assessing illiterate patients should be familiar with their normal function on psychometric tests. Psychological assessment of many migrant patients requires flexibility, creativity, and basic understanding (as opposed to "cookbook" acquaintance) of the evaluative process. The psychiatrist relying on psychological testing for migrant patients should know the psychologist's competence in the field, as well as the extent of culture-fairness of various tests for a particular patient. For example, patients familiar with paper and pencil should be able to perform the Porteus Maze well, whereas patients unfamiliar with pencil and paper may not perform on a par with their abilities. Timing in the course of the disorder is also critical. For example, a severely depressed migrant should not be assessed with a complete intelligence battery until the depression resolves (Draguns 1977; Nicassio et al. 1986).

Clinical rating scales based on psychiatric interview or psychiatric nursing observations can be useful to quantify the severity of the patient's condition (Hamilton 1967; Honigfeld and Klett 1965; Lou and Klett 1966; Overall and Gorham 1962). These scales allow the patient's condition to be assessed over time in order to determine treatment responsiveness or failure. Clinician-rated scales are especially valuable for psychiatric patients, since self-rating scales may not reflect the severity of the patient's condition as accurately as clinical rating scales (Prusoff et al. 1972; Winokur et al. 1982). Translating and restandardizing psychological tests and self-rating scales are expensive and time-consuming undertakings. Copies of numerous translated and restandardized tests can be obtained by writing the Refugee Assistance Program at the National Institute of Mental Health in Rockville, Maryland.

Autobiographies and drawings of traumatic events can aid migrant patients in telling their stories and expressing their perceptions and feelings. These techniques are applicable to patients in general, but are especially relevant for victims of traumatic experiences who may have difficulty expressing themselves in the usual face-to-face clinical setting. Children and adolescents are also good candidates for these facilitating methods (Carlin 1979).

Laboratory testing for organic brain damage, endocrine abnormalities, malnutrition, and parasitosis is especially important for migrant patients. Extensive life change, premigration crises, migration stresses, and postmigration challenges put them at high risk to various biomedical disorders. A routine test battery may need to be developed for particular migrant groups (e.g., ova and stool for parasites, urine drug screens). Certain tests, such as the electroencephalogram, require orientation and education for many migrants, such as those who have been tortured with electricity or who have no knowledge of the test methods or purposes (Brozek 1978; Winiek 1980).

Special Patient Subgroups

Age affects the assessment of migrants in a fashion similar for nonmigrants. However, there are some special issues that must be considered. Organic brain damage must be considered in migrant patients of all ages. Acquired brain damage in children, rarely seen in children born in the United States, is considerably more common in children exposed to war, civil unrest, malnutrition, and infectious disease. Physical mistreatment, torture, head beatings, infectious disease damage, and malnutrition may not produce clinical symptoms for decades until the person reaches 50 or 60 years of age, when other illnesses or aging amplify the earlier damage (Brozek 1978; Winiek 1980).

Environmental and social problems also differ with age. Children and adolescents may be exposed to racism, ethnic prejudice, or intergenerational stresses. They are also apt to experience abuse, neglect, or apathy from parents who have depression, PTSD, or other psychiatric disorders (Carlin 1979; Kremer and Sabin 1985). The elderly are more apt to suffer from social and cultural isolation, boredom, loss of social role and status, concerns about funereal practices and burial in a foreign land, and the obvious loss of their culture in their progeny. Inability to acquire language and lack of a work role in a new country can contribute to isolation and the risk to depression in the elderly, as well as in younger people who are illiterate, learning disabled, or intellectually impaired (Kiefer et al. 1986; Nicassio et al. 1986).

Migrants manifest age-related modifications in psychopathology similar to those observed in nonmigrants. For example, depressed children and adolescents are more apt to manifest hypersomnia, absence from school, falling grades, problems in social relationships with peers and authority figures, sports injuries, drug abuse, feigned illness, hyperactivity, aggressiveness, and nihilism. Elderly depressed persons are more apt to manifest confusion, memory loss, poor grooming, intellectual deterioration, and exacerbation of chronic medical conditions (e.g., diabetes, hypertension, congestive heart disease). However, cultural differences in age-appropriate behavior can lead to misdiagnosis if psychiatrists are unfamiliar with them (Kiefer et al. 1986; Kremer and Sabin 1985).

Sex also affects assessment of migrants in ways typical of nonmigrants, but with a few special considerations. Male migrants are more apt to have lost traditional occupations, avocations, roles, and statuses. These losses should be reviewed, along with efforts and successes in replacing these since migration. Women are at risk to emotional neglect or physical abuse from depressed or paranoid husbands or boyfriends. Robbery, assault, and rape are also more apt to occur among female migrants compared to male migrants. Women accustomed to homebound or village-bound work are apt to experience social phobias and anxiety in association with employment away from the immediate home environment (Rumbaut and Rumbaut 1976; Westermeyer et al. 1983b).

Sex affects psychopathology in migrants much as in nonmigrants. For example, depressed women are more apt to feel and look sad, blame themselves, have crying spells, and consider suicide. Depressed men are more apt to feel and look angry, blame others, have temper tantrums, abuse substances, and consider assault or homicide.

Socioeconomic status (SES) prior to migration can affect assessment in various ways. Especially if a bilingual worker or psychiatric interpreter is involved, class, education, or urban/rural differences can intrude on the patient-interpreter relationship. Patients may feel inferior to or demeaned by a formerly "higher class" interpreter. Interpreters can also encounter countertransference feelings toward patients of different class backgrounds. These transference and countertransference feelings can be even more disruptive if patient and interpreter belong to different ethnic groups from the same country. Those of like cultural background and language, but from different countries, can also encounter problems in working together clinically, due to old prejudices and stereotypes.

Class problems may be manifest in many languages that have class and "respect" terms built into the language. In some languages it is virtually impossible to avoid class/respect terminology. For example, the Lao language has several personal pronouns for "I, you, he, they" depending on relative status. Terms for "I" also include the following:

gu: for speaking to children, formerly used in addressing slaves, infers "talking down";
coy: used among friends and family, infers an equalitarian relationship;
kha-noi: literally "I a little slave," used in addressing older or higher class or respected persons;
kha-pha-tschow: literally "I the slave of the Buddha," used in formal public address to a group;
kha-pha-phat: abbreviated form of "I the slave of the sole of the foot of the king," used only in addressing royalty.

In clinical settings, interpreters should be aware that formal and respectful terms should ordinarily be employed with adults, especially older people. Children and adolescents are more comfortable with less formal terms of address.

Victims of terror, torture, combat, prison or concentration camps, starvation or malnutrition, forced work, prolonged exposure to the elements, and refugee flight require more intensive and extensive assessment than most psychiatric patients. Symptoms of PTSD must be reviewed directly and explicitly; spontaneous reporting by the patient cannot be assumed. Mental status and neurological examinations (including such "soft signs" as frontal lobe signs and incoordination) should be conducted, along with a routine physical exam and screening laboratory tests. Special brain imaging and testing may be needed, including X-ray, electroencephalography, nuclear magnetic resonance (NMR) imaging, or various psychological tests. Extensive interviewing of the patients concerning violent or stressful events should be undertaken by those who will conduct the treatment, so that patients are not repeatedly subjected to the distress of reporting these events.

Family assessment, always important in psychiatric assessment, looms even larger for migrants for several reasons (Rumbaut and Rumbaut 1976). Marital and intergenerational conflicts are often present in these cases. In many societies the family rather than the individual makes decisions regarding medical assessment or treatment, so that knowledge about and a relationship with the family often affects treatment compliance and outcome. In some cases the patient cannot be treated independently of the family unit, as when a depressed wife is being physically abused by a husband. Family relationships are often intensified for a period of months following migration, so that family often functions as pathogen or treatment resource (or both) even more strongly than in nonmigrant families. In the case of unaccompanied refugee children, adopted immigrant children, and cross-racially adopted children presenting for treatment, family assessment often presents unique challenges (Shuval et al. 1967, Sorosky et al. 1975).

Diagnostic Categories and Systems

Cultural differences in psychiatric systems and categories cause less mischief in the real clinical world than inadequate skill, information, and time taken in conducting psychiatric assessment of migrants. Nonetheless, the history of psychiatric diagnoses and classification systems is relevant to assessment of migrants. This history informs us regarding the impressive diagnostic advances in psychiatry, their application across cultures and languages (given careful assessment procedures), and the need for high diagnostic skill in those caring for migrants. As will be emphasized in the following section on psychodynamics and sociodynamics, descriptive psychopathological diagnoses by themselves are incomplete for adequate treatment planning and rehabilitation in many, perhaps most, cases. At the same time, careful descriptive diagnosis (and repeated diagnostic reassessment over time) is critical to appropriate management and optimal outcome. Neither diagnostic nor dynamic thinking should be replaced by the other; both are necessary.

Kraepelin observed around 1900 that "our clinical concepts vary so widely that for the foreseeable future such comparison is possible only if the observations are made by one and the same observer" (Kraepelin 1904). A half century later, Galdstone (1957) affirmed a "national psychiatry" in various countries, yet lamented the absence of an international psychiatry in the same sense that there was an international surgery. Three decades since then an international psychiatry has been evolving. One factor in this evolution has been the development of new and effective pharmacotherapies (e.g., tricyclics, monoamine oxidase inhibitors, lithium, neuroleptics) and psychotherapies (e.g., desensitization for phobias, cognitive therapy for chronic depressions, token economy systems for mental retardation, contingency contracting for behavioral disorders). These new therapies have aided in validating diagnostic categories based on treatment responsiveness. These effective new therapies, largely starting during the 1950s, led to greater efforts in qualifying and quantifying psychopathology. Overall and Gorham (1962), Klett along with co-workers Lou and Honigfield (Honigfield and Klett 1965, Lou and Klett 1966), and Hamilton (1967) initiated efforts during the 1960s aimed at symptom-level description based on psychiatric interview. Empirically developed psychometrics and standardization across languages and cultures (such as the MMPI) have also contributed to the evolution of reliable diagnostic categories during the 1970s and 1980s (Butcher and Pancheri 1976; Butcher and Spielberger 1985; Brislin 1970). Based on this infrastructure the St. Louis and Iowa groups developed research criteria for diagnostic entities that were widely accepted. This eventuated in the work of Spitzer and others in developing the strongly symptom-based third edition of the *Diagnostic and Statistical Manual of Mental Disorders* (DSM-III) by the American Psychiatric Association. As this is written, the World Health Organization (WHO) is undertaking a similar modification of the psychiatric categories in the *International Classification of Diseases* for its tenth edition (ICD-10). International efforts for diagnostic standards have been promulgated by Sartorius and Jablensky of WHO working with several English investigators, as well as with collaborators from all regions of the world (Cooper et al. 1969; Sartorius et al. 1980).

Studies of cross-cultural and cross-language diagnosis have also advanced the reliability of psychiatric diagnosis across ethnic and national boundaries. Perceptive analysts have addressed the semantic (Collomb 1965), philosophical (Kroll 1979), and categorical (Lachman 1970) issues involving international diagnostic schemata. These reports have shown the extent to which national values, as well as culture-related content and behavioral styles in psychopathology can affect diagnostic practice. Since 1970, comparative studies of diagnostic practices among psychiatrists from different countries have also been valuable in identifying idiosyncratic national preferences in order to bring these into conformity with international practice (Cooper et al. 1969; Kendell et al. 1971; Surawicz and Sandifer 1970; Westermeyer and Sines 1979). Work in this area now continues at several centers around the world.

Folk syndromes are infrequently encountered in psychiatric settings, even in countries where they have been described. Examples include *amok* (sudden and sometimes indiscriminate homicidal assaults), *latah* (explosive yelling, often of curses or vulgar expressions), *koro* (fear of genital shrinkage and possible death), and "cardiac neurosis" or "nervous breakdown" in the United States. Although they are not common clinical entities among migrants, they do occur and can create confusion if clinicians are not prepared for them. One erroneous notion is that they are distinct clinical or psychiatric syndromes, with their own etiologies, courses, treatments, prognoses, and outcomes. In fact, they tend to be common behavioral manifestations that are associated with diverse psychiatric diagnoses. For example, *amok* and *latah* can be associated with personality disorders, adjustment disorders, substance abuse, major depression, mania, organic brain syndromes, and schizophrenia (Ben-Tovim 1985; Friedman and Faguet 1982; Westermeyer 1973). A second error is to assume that a folk therapist (rather than a psychiatrist) should necessarily assume care of the patient with a folk syndrome. Those migrants presenting to psychiatric facilities with folk syndromes should receive the usual psychiatric evaluation being employed for other migrant

101

patients. A third problem is that clinicians and other gatekeepers tend to underrate the severity of the clinical problem, suggesting that it is "traditional" and therefore trivial. An example is opium addiction among recent Southeast Asian refugees in the United States, which is as fully morbid a condition as heroin addiction among native-born Americans.

Personality disorders (i.e., Axis II of the DSM-III system) present particular problems in the diagnosis of migrants, especially if cross-cultural diagnosis is involved. Careful evaluation of Axis II diagnosis in 109 Cuban refugees revealed a high rate of unconfirmed and probably erroneous diagnoses (Boxer and Garvey 1985). Of course, considerable difference in opinion, reliability problems, and lack of validity data exists even for intracultural personality diagnoses. Migration can exacerbate personality disorders. Certain personality types may retard the process of acculturation or social adaptation. For example, shy, overly dependent, or paranoid personalities may pose special risks to the migrant's adjustment (Boxer and Garvey 1985). The following information assists in detecting the presence or absence of personality disorder: the patient's level of adjustment, interpersonal relationships, and social competence prior to migration; the patient's previous ability to cope with loss, extensive life change, and major stressors; the patient's previous ability to form attachments, and obtain and maintain a normal-sized social network; and prior to migration, patient's ability to set goals, make commitments, implement plans, and achieve objectives.

Personality disorder diagnoses should not be readily made in migrants, at least for a period of time after migration and for a time after treatment has been instituted. This is especially true in refugees, torture victims, and prisoners of war who are apt to manifest transient characteristics of personality disorder (Sack et al. 1986). Passive dependence or passive aggressiveness may be acquired personality styles that were adaptive in the refugee or concentration camp, and perhaps previously under repressive political regimes.

PTSD can mimic personality disorder through the avoidance of close interpersonal relationships and emotional "numbing" that are often associated with this syndrome. Organic personality disorder may occur in those veterans, refugees, and others with brain damage. Paranoid personality disorders may appear for the first time after a migration.

Psychodynamics and Sociodynamics

With experience and supervision, psychiatrists readily acquire skill and self-confidence in making descriptive DSM-III-R diagnoses. However, the ability to assess dynamically tends to take longer. This longer learning curve to attain dynamic assessment skills is largely due to unfamiliarity with a range of cultures. Once the clinician is familiar with a range of foreign students, returning combat veterans, family members of migrant executives or seasonal workers, refugees, and others, the ability to recognize and explore psychological and social dynamic issues becomes second nature.

Making merely a descriptive diagnosis is similar to making a biomedical diagnosis of congestive heart failure without considering the individual pathophysiology in the case. For biomedical disease, pathophysiological analysis is necessary in order to ascertain etiology (e.g., anemia, hyperthyroidism, beriberi, coronary artery disease, hypertensive heart disease) so that effective treatment and rehabilitation can be implemented (including heading off subsequent recurrences, e.g., of congestive heart failure). Similarly, the rationales for making a psychopathological analysis of the case, including both a descriptive diagnosis and analysis of the psychological and social dynamics, are: to ascertain the etiology of the disorder, including the severity of the losses or stressors vis-à-vis the vulnerability of the individual; to identify factors that are apt to produce recurrences if not addressed (e.g., through psychotherapy, family counseling, acculturation counseling, milieu change, education); to determine whether there are ongoing factors that cannot be modified, so as to assess the degree of chronic vulnerability; to devise the most effective treatment alternatives; and to maximize compliance.

In order to appreciate psychodynamics and sociodynamics among migrants, the clinician must be familiar with materials in earlier chapters. These include concepts such as the developmental aspects of ensocialization, social network loss and reconstruction, "technology shock," "culture shock," acculturation, and acculturative stress. Factors leading to aversive or biased migration (whether political, economic, family, or individually determined) should be appreciated. Since some migrants have been victimized before, during, or after their migration, the psychiatrist must be cognizant of the common dynamic issues among assault and rape victims, those tortured by the enemy versus by their own people, and survivors of battle or disaster. Culture and ethnicity can determine both psychodynamics and sociodynamics to a considerable extent, so that an awareness of culture factors in general is important, along with more individualized knowledge of the patient's own particular ethnic behavioral and ideal norms, attitudes, customs, affiliations, and traditionality.

References

Bazzouli W, Al-Issa I: Psychiatry in Iraq. Br J Psychiatry 112:827–832, 1966

Benedict PK, Jacks J: Mental illness in primitive societies. Psychiatry 17:377–389, 1954

Ben-Tovim DI: DSM-III in Botswana: a field trial in a developing country. Am J Psychiatry 142:342–345, 1985

Berkanovic E: The effect of inadequate language translation on Hispanic's responses to health surveys. Am J Public Health 70:1273–1276, 1980

Boleloucky Z, Horwath M: SCL-90 rating scales: first experience with the Czech version in healthy male scientific workers. Activitas Nervosa Superior (Prague) 16:115–116, 1974

Boxer DA, Garvey JT: Psychiatric diagnoses of Cuban refugees in the United States: findings of medical review boards. Am J Psychiatry 142:86–89, 1985

Brislin RW: Back translation for cross-cultural research. Journal of Cross-Cultural Psychology 1:185–216, 1970

Brozek J: Nutrition, malnutrition, and behavior. Annu Rev Psychol 29:157–177, 1978

Butcher JN, Garcia R: Cross-national application of psychological tests. Personnel and Guidance 56:472–475, 1978

Butcher JN, Gur R: A Hebrew translation of the MMPI: an assessment of translation adequacy and preliminary validation. Journal of Cross-Cultural Psychology 5:220–227, 1974

Butcher JN, Pancheri P: A Handbook of Cross National MMPI Research. Minneapolis, University of Minnesota Press, 1976

Butcher JN, Spielberger CD: Advances in Personality Assessment, Vol 4. Hillsdale, NJ, Earlbaum Press, 1985

Carlin JE: Southeast Asian refugee children, in Basic Handbook of Child Psychiatry, Vol 1. Edited by Nospitz JD, Call JD, Cohen RL, Berlin IH. New York, Basic Books, 1979, pp 290–300

Chien CC: Application of self rating symptoms to psychiatric out-patients. Bulletin of the Chinese Society of Neurology and Psychiatry 4:47–56, 1978

Cochrane R, Hashmi F, Stopes-Roe M: Measuring psychological disturbance in Asian immigrants to Britain. Soc Sci Med 11:157–164, 1977

Collomb M: Boufees delirantes en psychiatrie Africaine. Psychopathologie Africaine 1:167–239, 1965

Cooper JE, Kendall RE, Gurland BJ, et al: Cross-national study of diagnosis of mental disorders: some results from the first comparative investigation. Am J Psychiatry (April Suppl) 125:21–29, 1969

DelCastillo JC: The influence of language upon symptomatology in foreign-born patients. Am J Psychiatry 127:242–244, 1970

Derogatis LR, Covi L, Lipman RS, et al: Social class and race as mediator variables in neurotic symptomatology. Arch Gen Psychiatry 25:31–40, 1971

Derogatis LR, Lipman RS, Covi L: SCL-90: an outpatient psychiatric rating scale—preliminary report. Psychopharmacol Bull 9:13–28, 1973

Draguns J: Advances in the methodology of cross-cultural psychiatric assessment. Transcultural Psychiatric Research Review 14:125–143, 1977

Edgerton RB, Karno M: Mexican-American bilingualism and the perception of mental illness. Arch Gen Psychiatry 24:286–290, 1971

El-Islam MF, Malasi TH: Delusions and education. Journal of Operational Psychiatry 16:29–31, 1985

El Sendiony HFM: Cultural aspects of delusions: a psychiatry study of Egypt. Aust N Z J Psychiatry 10:201–207, 1976

Escobar JI, Burman A, Karno M, et al: Use of the Mini-Mental Status Examination (MMSE) in a community population of mixed ethnicity. J Nerv Ment Dis 174:607–614, 1986

Fleiss JL: Statistical Methods for Rates and Proportions. New York, Wiley, 1973

Friedman CTH, Faguet R: Extraordinary Disorders of Human Behavior. New York, Plenum, 1982

Galdstone I: International psychiatry. Am J Psychiatry 114:103–108, 1957

Goodenough WH: Ethnographic field techniques, in Handbook of Cross-Cultural Psychology. Edited by Triandis HC, Berry JW. Boston, Allyn Bacon, 1980

Hall ET: The Silent Language. Garden City, NY, Doubleday, 1959

Hamilton W: Development of a rating scale for primary depressive illness. British Journal of Social and Clinical Psychology 6:278–296, 1967

Honigfield G, Klett CJ: The Nurse's Observation Scale for Inpatient Evaluation (NOSIE): a new scale for measuring improvement in chronic schizophrenia. J Clin Psychol 21:65–71, 1965

Kendell RE, Cooper JE, Gourlay AJ, et al: Diagnostic criteria of American and British psychiatrists. Arch Gen Psychiatry 25:122–130, 1971

Kiefer CW, Kim S, Chai K, et al: Adjustment problems of Korean American elderly. Gerontologist 25:477–482, 1986

Kim KI, Won HT, Lee JH, et al: Standardization study of Symptom Checklist-90 in Korea, I: characteristics of normal responses. Journal of the Korean Neuropsychiatric Association 17:449–458, 1978

Kinzie JD, Manson SM: The use of self-rating scales in cross-cultural psychiatry. Hosp Community Psychiatry 38:190–196, 1987

Kinzie JD, Manson SM, Vinh DT, et al: Development and validation of a Vietnamese-language depression rating scale. Am J Psychiatry 139:1276–1281, 1982

Klaf FS, Hamilton JG: Schizophrenia—a hundred years ago and today. Journal of Mental Science 107:276–283, 1973

Kline F, Acosta FX, Austin W, et al: The misunderstood Spanish-speaking patient. Am J Psychiatry 137:1530–1533, 1980

Kraepelin E: Lectures on Clinical Psychiatry. Edited by Johnstone F. New York, William Wood, 1904

Kremer PG, Sabin C: Indochinese immigrant children: problems in psychiatric diagnosis. J Am Acad Child Psychiatry 2:453–458, 1985

Kroll J: Philosophical foundations of French and U.S. nosology. Am J Psychiatry 136:1135–1138, 1979

Lachman JH: Swedish and American psychiatry: a comparative view. Am J Psychiatry 126:1777–1781, 1970

Leff JP: Transcultural influences on psychiatrists' rating of verbally expressed emotion. Br J Psychiatry 125:336–340, 1974

Lieblich I, Kugelmmass S, Ben-Shakhar G: Psychophysiological baselines as a function of race and ethnic origin. Psychopathology 10:426–430, 1973

Lin KM, Tazuma L, Masuda M: Adaptational problems of

Vietnamese refugees, I: health and mental health status. Arch Gen Psychiatry 36:955–961, 1979

Lou M, Klett CJ: Inpatient Multidimensional Psychiatric Scale. Palo Alto, CA, Consulting Psychologist Press, 1966

Marcos LR: Effects of interpreters on the evaluation of psychopathology in non-English-speaking patients. Am J Psychiatry 136:171–174, 1979

Marcos LR, Urcuyo L, Kesselman M, et al: The language barrier in evaluating Spanish-American patients. Arch Gen Psychiatry 29:655–659, 1973

Nicassio PM, Solomon GS, Guest SS, et al: Emigration stress and language proficiency as correlates of depression in a sample of Southeast Asian refugees. Int J Soc Psychiatry 32:22–28, 1986

Nichter M: Idioms of distress, alternatives in the expression of psychosocial distress: a case history from South India. Cult Med Psychiatry 3:379–408, 1981

Opler MK: Cultural differenes in mental disorders: an Italian and Irish contrast in the schizophrenias—USA, in Culture and Mental Health. Edited by Opler MK. New York, Macmillan, 1959, pp 425–442

Overall JE, Gorham DR: The Brief Psychiatric Rating Scale. Psychol Rep 10:799-812, 1962

Peck EC: The relationship of disease and other stress to second language. Int J Soc Psychiatry 20:128–133, 1974

Prusoff BA, Klerman GL, Paykel ES: Concordance between clinical assessments and patients' self report in depression. Arch Gen Psychiatry 16:546–552, 1972

Rumbaut RE, Rumbaut RG: The family in exile: Cuban expatriates in the United States. Am J Psychiatry 133:395–399, 1976

Sabin JE: Translating despair. Am J Psychiatry 132:197–199, 1975

Sack WH, Angell RH, Kinzie JD, et al: The psychiatric effects of massive trauma on Cambodian children, II: the family, the home, the school. J Am Acad Child Psychiatry 25:377–383, 1986

Sartorius N, Jablensky A, Gulbinat W, et al: Preliminary communication, WHO collaborative study: assessment of depressive disorders. Psychol Med 10:743–749, 1980

Shuval JT, Antonovsky A, Davies DM: The doctor-patient relationship in an ethnically heterogeneous society. Soc Sci Med 1:141–154, 1967

Simons RC, Hughes CC (eds): The Culture-Bound Syndromes: Folk Illnesses of Psychiatric and Anthropological Interest. Boston, Reidel Publishing, 1985

Sorosky A, Baran A, Pannon R: Identity conflicts in adoptees. Am J Orthopsychiatry 45:18–27, 1975

Spiegel JP: Cultural aspects of transference and countertransference revisited. J Am Acad Psychoanal 4:447–467, 1976

Steinbrunner S, Scharfetter C: Changes in delusional psychosis— a historical transcultural comparison. Archiv fur Psychiatrie and Nervenkrankheitan 222:47–60, 1976

Surawicz FG, Sandifer MG: Cross cultural diagnosis: a study of psychiatric diagnosis, comparing Switzerland, the United States, and the United Kingdom. Int J Soc Psychiatry 16:232–236, 1970

Tyhurst L: Displacement and migration: a study in social psychiatry. Am J Psychiatry 107:561–566, 1951

Uchigama K, Lutterjohn M, Shah MD: Crosscultural differences in frontalis muscle tension levels: an exploratory study comparing Japanese and Westerners. Biofeedback Self Regul 6:75–78, 1981

Weinstein EA: Cultural Aspects of Delusions. New York, Free Press, 1962

Westermeyer J: On the epidemicity of amok. Arch Gen Psychiatry 28:873–876, 1973

Westermeyer J: Psychiatric diagnoses across cultural boundaries. Am J Psychiatry 142:798–805, 1985

Westermeyer J: Two self rating scales for depression in Hmong refugees: assessment in clinical and nonclinical samples. J Psychiatr Res 20:103–113, 1986

Westermeyer J: Clinical considerations in cross cultural diagnosis. Hosp Community Psychiatry 38:160–165, 1987a

Westermeyer J: Cultural factors in clinical assessment. J Consult Clin Psychol 55:471–478, 1987b

Westermeyer J: Some cross cultural aspects of delusions, in Delusional Beliefs. Edited by Oltmanns T, Maher BA. New York, Wiley, 1988, pp 212–229

Westermeyer J, Sines L: Reliability of cross-cultural psychiatric diagnoses with an assessment of two rating contexts. J Psychiatr Res 15:199–213, 1979

Westermeyer J, Zimmerman R: Lao folk diagnoses for mental disorder: comparison with psychiatric diagnoses and assessment with psychiatric rating scales. Med Anthropol 5:425–443, 1981

Westermeyer J, Vang TF, Neider J: A comparison of refugees using and not using a psychiatric service: an analysis of DSM-III criteria and self-rating scales in cross-cultural context. J Operational Psychiatry 14:36–41, 1983a

Westermeyer J, Vang TF, Neider J: Hmong refugees in Minnesota: characteristics and self perceptions. Minn Med 66:431–439, 1983b

Winiek M: Nutrition and brain development. Natural History 89:6–13, 1980

Winkelmayer R, Gottheil E, Exline RV, et al: The relative accuracy of U.S., British, and Mexican raters in judging the emotional displays of schizophrenic and normal U.S. women. J Clin Psychol 34:600–608, 1978

Winokur A, Guthrie MB, Rickels K, et al: Extent of agreement between patient and physician ratings of emotional distress. Psychosomatics 23:1135–1146, 1982

Wittkower ED, Murphy HB, Fried J, et al: A cross-cultural inquiry into the symptomatology of schizophrenia. Ann NY Acad Sci 84:854–863, 1960

Zung WWF: A self-rating depression scale. Arch Gen Psychiatry 12:63–70, 1975

Chapter 5
Clinical Management

Chapter 5

Clinical Management

Developing a treatment plan for migrant patients may seem, at first glance, to be an impossible task. Understanding cultural differences, the immediate and long-term goals, working with interpreters, and other conceptual and logistical problems can make clinical care for these patients appear overwhelming. Although psychiatric care of immigrants does tend to be more time consuming and complicated (at least initially), it is well within the abilities of most well-trained, reasonably sensitive, and fairly creative psychiatrists. The key lies in simplifying the process. Basically, the clinician's usual procedures and best judgment must be applied, with allowances for the particular circumstances of the case at hand.

The first step, as in any case, involves completing a thorough assessment. Once the patient is well known and the diagnosis is established, treatment planning evolves naturally in a way familiar to the psychiatrist. Confusion regarding clinical management usually results from an inadequate assessment. As treatment proceeds, repeated reassessment is critical in evaluating treatment efforts to date and in guiding future treatment efforts. Failure of the usual treatment is an indication for a complete reassessment, possibly including consultation by a cultural psychiatrist and/or a cultural psychologist.

This chapter aims at helping the psychiatrist to undertake a management plan. This undertaking requires appropriate goal setting and treatment planning, recognition of the patient's views and expectations, and knowledge of special clinical and logistical dilemmas apt to occur among migrant patients. Success in the care of these patients inevitably produces positive attitudes in the clinician, so that further work with such patients ensues.

Goals of Treatment

For acute problems with a favorable outcome and a brief course, the usual goal is amelioration of the patient's condition. Success in overcoming their problems in foreign locations can greatly contribute to patients' self-esteem and maturation. Returning home prematurely, without the goal of the migration accomplished, can create a long lasting self-image (as well as social image) as a failure. Migrant patients can look quite ill in cross-section. However, if their symptoms have been present for a short period and a crisis event can be identified, response to treatment can be rapid and complete.

The clinician must sometimes counsel and support the patient and family during the time-consuming process of adaptation and acculturation in the new society. Crisis reactions, nightmares and temper tantrums in refugee children, regression in relocated adolescents, and family and generational conflict can often be effectively reversed by a modicum of patient guidance and warm empathy. While major psychopathology is often present in the migrant reaching psychiatric facilities, it is not always present (Sokoloff et al. 1984) but may ensue if migrant cases are mishandled.

In other cases, the immediate goal of treatment is sufficient alleviation of symptoms to allow the patient to travel home. The person may have been about to travel home anyway, or the severity of the illness may warrant a return to resources closer to home. Readiness of the patient to return home is a critical decision. At times a decision must be made that the patient must be accompanied on the journey home, perhaps by family, professionals, or both.

The following circumstances may lead to return home or repatriation:

- The patient had a chronic disorder before migration and is returning home for ongoing care;
- Adequate finances to pay for the patient's ongoing care are not available in the new community;
- Despite adequate care, the patient continues to have continuous or recurrent symptoms in association with acculturation stress and/or acculturation failure.

The goal of returning home versus remaining in the current community may not be readily apparent at the time of assessment. However, it usually becomes apparent within the first few weeks of hospital care, or the first several weeks of outpatient care. As a general rule, patients who have already acculturated well to the new setting do well enough to remain while completing school, visiting relatives, or continuing work. Those who have become severely disabled within days or weeks of arrival (i.e., before having acculturated), or have not acculturated despite many months or years in the new residence, usually must be repatriated. Patients whose illnesses are refractory to treatment, even though they have acculturated to a partial extent, probably should return home. In such cases, their prognosis is typically improved by a return to family, a familiar culture, and local resources.

Even in circumstances favoring a return home, this may not always be a viable alternative. Refugees, asylum seekers, and politically displaced persons are a case in point, since return home may result in imprisonment, or even execution. Those displaced by dam construction, atomic tests, chemical accidents, volcanic eruptions, and other disasters may similarly be unable to return to their familiar origins. Other migrants could theoretically return home, but economic forces augur against it. This group consists of workers from economically depressed areas, executives or government workers transferred by their employers, and American Indians from reservations that have high unemployment. Noneconomic considerations preventing a return home include the desire for training and education, wanting to remain with a spouse or family, and unwillingness to leave a valued new community or life-style. In these cases the clinician must attempt to aid the patient in resettling while concurrently dealing with the associated psychiatric problem—not a simple task.

For the patient who has become ill before acculturating, yet cannot return home, goal setting should include a reasonable level of adjustment and/or acculturation. Adaptation to a different culture or adjustment to a new community is difficult for a person who is concurrently trying to deal with recovery from depression, social phobia, or other disorder. Acculturation may necessarily be incomplete in patients with certain chronic disorders that are even partially disabling, such as schizophrenia, mental retardation, or organic brain syndromes.

Nowadays one occasionally hears that the goal of an intervention may be to treat the patient's combat, "torture," or other traumatic experience. All victims of torture, combat, persecution, and other forms of victimization do not develop PTSD or other psychiatric disorders (Kinzie and Fleck 1987)—just as all children surviving psychotic or alcoholic parents do not emerge from their childhoods with stress, loss, and trauma. It is not at all clear that treatment of nonsymptomatic victims is warranted. As Kinzie and co-workers (Kinzie 1985; Kinzie and Fleck 1987) have pointed out, well-intentioned but amateurish, nonindicated, or poorly timed interventions can precipitate or exacerbate psychopathology. Anecdotal case histories suggest that many people cope with these past events through their own grief work, cultural ceremonies, religious rituals, informal group support, and anniversary gatherings with fellow survivors—repeating these rituals and ceremonies at intervals through the remainder of their lives. At this point we do not know whether therapy in nonsymptomatic victims can reduce their vulnerability to a subsequent psychiatric disorder or enhance their psychosocial functioning. There may be value in making a period of education, ventilation, or group support available to symptomatic but not necessarily disabled persons soon after rape, torture, combat, terrorist hostage taking, and similar experiences (Masters et al. 1988; Roth and Lebowitz 1988). Brief intervention of this sort should not substitute for psychiatric assessment and care in cases with persisting or disabling symptoms. Hopefully, controlled studies in this area will guide further treatment and prevention planning.

Treatment Planning

Generally the treatment planning for migrant patients resembles that of other patients. Diagnosis, psychodynamic and sociodynamic factors, treatment alternatives, and treatment resources determine planning to a considerable extent. However, several additional factors also influence planning in the case of migrants.

One of these factors concerns sociotherapies, such as acculturation, employment rehabilitation, language training, and social-network reconstruction. These are dealt with in a subsequent chapter in more detail. If the patient needs them in order to adjust to the new society but they are not available, this argues for a return to the community of origin. If the patient requires them and they are available, then cooperation with the programs providing them is necessary. A double-bind situation can intrude here. For example, social or educational agencies may say that they cannot work with the patient until he or she is completely recovered from a psychiatric disorder; but in order to recover completely from the psychiatric disorder the patient needs to have social and educational services. Another common problem is that vocational services will not provide help until the patient speaks English, but most migrants do not acquire a working knowledge of English until they are in a regular job or an integrated school setting. In order to surmount these systems obstacles, considerable administrative time must be devoted to laying the groundwork for cooperation.

Involvement of the bilingual psychiatric worker in the treatment plan is crucial for patients who do not speak the psychiatrist's language or are from another culture. This worker is usually responsible for implementing certain aspects of the plan, explaining it to the patient, negotiating details of the plan between patient and clinician, and making follow-up contacts to ensure implementation of the plan. Consequently, the bilingual worker must appreciate the goals, elements, and potential problems associated with the treatment plan. Depending on the psychiatric training and experience of the worker, this critical step may demand little extra time, or very considerable extra time. Even if just a psychiatrist and bilingual worker are involved on the case, a team approach to management is warranted. This team approach requires extra communication, clarification regarding each person's respective responsibilities, and regular meetings of the treatment team so as to head off misunderstanding.

Other helpers besides the treatment team are involved in the care of migrants. These others can include school counselors, teachers, other physicians, agency workers, police, correction or probation workers, the courts, immigration officials, and psychiatrists working elsewhere. This structure adds to the time and complexity of working out a treatment plan, but without this added effort, the plan is apt not to go well and the patient's recovery is impeded.

Management of the return or repatriation of the patient to the original community requires careful planning. The patient must be well enough to travel under psychiatric supervision. Airlines (the usual carrier by which repatriation is accomplished) require notification and clinical information ahead of time. Airline medical departments then consider the clinical data prior to giving their approval. Ordinarily first-class seats are required for purposes of room and airline staff must be available, in case these are needed. One person, usually a psychiatrist or nurse, must attend the patient. On long trips, two attendants can be required (only one need be a psychiatrist). If the patient has already been discharged from a hospital setting and is doing well, these strictures (i.e., approval, first-class seats, psychiatric attendants) may not be imposed. Family members may be deemed sufficient. Travel itself can exacerbate

118

psychiatric symptoms, however. Thus, it is best to err on the conservative side in arranging travel.

Two other arrangements must also be made prior to international travel. One of these is to contact the patient's embassy in order to alert them to the case, since immigration officials in the country of origin must be forewarned. If they are not, there may be inordinate delays upon reaching the country of origin. Ordinarily the Immigration and Naturalization Service can make these arrangements. Second, clinical facilities in the receiving country must be informed about the patient's return in order to ensure continuity of care. Notification usually can be arranged through the patient's embassy.

Psychiatric assessment and treatment may rely heavily on the family. Since kinship ties can vary widely from one ethnic group to another, clinicians should not ascribe their own kinship system to patients. To be sure, the European-based system of law in North America eventually influences the family organization of immigrants to a considerable extent. However, kinship systems do continue for decades and can continue through generations (Dunnigan 1982). Caught between cultures, some people may have difficulty in managing both the legal restrictions of society at large and the added extra-legal restrictions of their own ethnic group.

Culture Gap Between Patient and Psychiatrist

Ordinarily the migrant patient has little notion regarding the psychiatrist's scientific, as well as cultural knowledge and assumptions. While psychiatrists usually appreciate their own professional knowledge as psychiatrists, they are generally unaware of their own cultural norms, values, and attitudes. Similarly, patients may be able to provide the clinician with information on their own conceptual models of health, illness, and psychosocial dysfunction; but they may not be able to specify their own cultural norms, values, and attitudes (Hoang and Erickson 1985; Muecke 1983).

Since conceptual models of health and dysfunction are generally accessible, they can and should be discussed in the first session or two. Patients can be queried regarding their own ideas about their name for the problem, its causes, prognosis, treatments in their own culture, its course, and other manifestations. Family notions about these same topics also can be obtained. Discovering the patient's and family's own perspectives of the current disorder contributes to an understanding of both their traditional and modern knowledge regarding psychiatric disorders (Clement 1982; Edgerton 1966; Westermeyer 1979c; Westermeyer and Wintrob 1979a). Demon possession and religious influences, once common in European societies (Kemp and Williams 1987; Kroll and Bachrach 1982), are still encountered today in various parts of the world, including rural and ghetto America where fundamentalist religious beliefs prevail (Kemp and Williams 1987; Kroll and Bachrach 1982; Ward and Beaubrun 1981).

At some point, the psychiatrist will also want to convey to the patient (and usually also the patient's family) the psychiatric diagnosis; causes, precipitants, or vulnerabilities leading to the disorder; prognosis; and recommended treatment. This process involves educating the patient and the family. Mutual awareness between patient and psychiatrist can benefit each. For example, the clinician can use the patient's conceptual models to aid in the therapy, and the patient can add the clinician's conceptual models to those already existent.

Educating patients regarding psychiatric disorder can present serious obstacles when clinician and patient come from different societies. Even well-educated persons from other countries may not have acquired concepts regarding neurotransmitters, hallucinations, ensocialization, or acculturation. Psychological terms, while commonly used in North America, may be entirely unfamiliar—e.g., paranoid, passive aggressive, obsessive compulsive. Since education requires building on concepts already present, the clinician may need to establish the patient's and family's fund of information about neurophysiology, neuroanatomy, neuropsychology, neuropharmacology, psychology, or sociology in order to build upon it. In this regard, a smattering of knowledge on ethnopsychology (i.e., concepts regarding person, thought, emotions, and behavior across ethnic groups) and ethnopsychiatry (i.e., concepts regarding psychiatric disorder and methods among various ethnic groups) can assist greatly in educating the patient regarding the clinical problem at hand, and alternatives for dealing with it (Clement 1982; Marsella and White 1982; Westermeyer 1979b; White and Marsella 1982). It is important to remember that all cultures have terms and concepts for madness or insanity (Murphy 1976; Westermeyer 1979b). Other terms widely encountered in various cultures parallel such psychiatric terms as mental retardation, personality disorder, and the American folk notion of a "nervous breakdown" (Clement 1982; Resner and Hartog 1970; Westermeyer 1979b). Psychiatrists must abandon any stereotyping of simpler cultures as being idyllic and devoid of psychiatric disorder—a notion that has been well debunked over the last few decades (Fabrega and Metzger 1968; Jones and de la Horne 1973; Leighton et al. 1963).

Cultural norms, values, and attitudes may present greater problems for both patient and psychiatrist, since these are largely out of awareness. Even though people often can report their ideal norms (i.e., that which their culture prescribes), their behavioral norms (i.e., that which people in a particular culture actually do) may not be so readily admitted—especially to someone from another culture. One's own values and attitudes are also largely unquestioned. Examples include such variables as preferred marriage partners, spiritual goals in life, personal priorities, and material strivings (Hoang and Erickson 1985). Patients may not readily divulge their values and attitudes to a psychiatrist who, by culture, ethnicity, nationality, education, religion, or class, is apt to have very different values and attitudes—at least until the patient can trust the psychiatrist and can discern the psychiatrist's respect for the norms, values, and attitudes of the patient's society. Migrants are apt to interpret psychiatric disorder as being due to, or equivalent with sin, character defects, crime, and punishment by supernatural powers (Miller 1984; Wallace 1959). Such beliefs can further reduce the likelihood that patients and families will readily divulge certain clinically relevant information.

Migrant patients should be informed regarding professional, social, legal, and ethical dimensions of the psychiatrist-patient role in the United States. In some societies, confidentiality and anonymity are not assumed; on the contrary, the patient may assume that any information reported to the clinician may end up in the hands of the family, other physicians, the police, or immigration officials. Tarasoff-type laws (Bernal Y Del Rio 1985) do not exist in most societies, so that the American psychiatrist may need to warn the patient about the need to inform others if, in the psychiatrist's opinion, risk to a specific person exists. Similarly, American notions regarding informed consent are not universal and can prove problematic. For example, patients from some cultures may interpret education regarding the potential risk of a treatment as an effort by the psychiatrist to convince the patient against the treatment (although the clinician may actually be recommending the treatment).

It is well to keep in mind that language and culture can influence the expression of psychiatric symptoms (D'Andre and Egan 1974). For example, English tends to have many words to express anxiety (e.g., tense, uptight, strung out, anxious) whereas a virtual paragraph of somatic and psychological experiences is needed to capture this experience in some Asian languages. By contrast, the Thai-Lao languages have many more words to express sadness, loss, or frustration, than does English (e.g., literally, feeling "euk" in the chest, "little-hearted," "lost-hearted," "fallen-hearted," "screaming-hearted," "soft/weak hearted"). Degree of emotional expressiveness can also vary among cultures. For example, "smiling depression" (i.e., psychotic or melancholic depressed persons with a fixed, plastic smile) was once common in the United States, especially among rural Americans from Northern and Western European national origins, who did not want to disturb others by expressing their personal anguish and misery. "Smiling depression," now infrequent in the United States, is seen regularly among migrants from Asia and various rural regions. It should similarly be kept in mind that universals also exist in human experience (e.g., birth, death, pain, euphoria, loss, gain, success, failure, love, hate, parents, offspring, friends, enemies) and in psychopathological signs and symptoms, and these are reflected in universal concepts (White 1980).

The clinician must avoid stereotyping patients and families. All of us bear part of our culture's traditional concepts, but none of us bears all of them. Differences may exist among family members as well. For example, the Afro-American wife of a psychotic African immigrant firmly believed that some local members of the black community, certain men in particular, had "worked roots" (i.e., done a curse using voodoo-like methods) on her husband. Her African-born husband thought that this was entirely untrue and had a quite different explanation for his problem. Intermarriage of partners from different cultures, as in this example, is more apt to result in such different viewpoints; but they can and do occur even among family members from the same culture (Westermeyer and Wintrob 1979b).

Management of Special Types of Patients

The solitary migrant patient presents to treatment alone, without family, friends, or other social resources. Typically, these patients have recently arrived as students, visitors, workers, or tourists. Their assessment can pose special problems, since collateral sources of information and a longitudinal history from others is not readily available. If the patient is a voluntary, cooperative, nonpsychotic outpatient, the assessment obstacles are less than if the patient is an involuntary, psychotic, uncooperative, potentially dangerous inpatient. Treatment of the solitary patient as an outpatient can also present serious problems if there is no one to monitor medications, provide companionship, alert the clinician to signs of recurrence, or otherwise assist in a recovery plan. This may lead to more prolonged hospitalization than might otherwise be the case.

Dangerous patients can also put the clinician in a difficult position. If the patient is alone, no family member or friend may be available to initiate commitment proceedings. In some cultures, the individual is viewed as having a "right" to commit suicide, even though distraught, intoxicated, or mentally ill when the suicide decision is made. Thus, the family may agree with the presence of suicide risk but refuse to initiate commitment. This may prove a difficult situation for clinicians, since an administrative commitment may go against the wishes of both the family and the patient. People caught between two cultures can also be victimized by differing societal values toward self-destruction.

Patients dangerous to others due to psychiatric disorder do not create so much family opposition to commitment. Still, the family may prefer to stand by in a neutral way, permitting an administrative commitment while not actively supporting it. No society has ready answers to these difficult problems, and—while many societies permit suicide—societies do not easily accept the slaughter of innocent people at the hands of a mentally ill person. Further complicating matters, the patient may be dangerous more due to cultural differences in expectation and legal differences, rather than to psychiatric disorder. For example, revenge killing may be culturally prescribed under certain circumstances.

The patient who is legally a minor (child or adolescent) may present special management problems (Deinard and Dunnigan 1987). One of these consists of the parents not wanting psychiatric care for a child, especially if the absence of such care is likely to affect the minor's lifelong adjustment. Child protection agencies, the police, and courts may become involved. Such cases have several origins, none of which are easily overcome. The family might be hiding the mentally ill child due to shame. Such attitudes are a holdover from cultures in which mental illness is felt to reflect moral inferiority in the family. Or the family may fear that the child would be taken away and never returned—a possible occurrence in some countries in which psychiatric care consists of long-term "warehousing" of the mentally ill in large, impersonal institutions. Families may provide young retardates or mentally ill persons with minimal care, with the expectation that death will ensue. Family members can be acculturating at different rates so that a division of opinion may exist within the family, with some members wanting psychiatric care and other members opting for traditional alternatives.

Cross-racial adoptees might be expected to be at lower risk to maladjustment or psychiatric disorder since their adoptive parents tend to be above average in terms of income, social stability, desire for children, and willingness to provide a good home. On the contrary, adopted children and adolescents have a higher-than-expected rate for many forms of psychopathology. This is probably due to a combination of genetic and intrauterine factors, and (sometimes) abuse or neglect during infancy. Cross-racial adoption often involves adoption of children with more pigment by parents of less pigment (and seldom the reverse). Thus, children can grow up with an acquired ethnic identity that does not match their racial inheritance. This can create serious identity problems during adolescence and early adulthood—a time of identity struggle and formation. This phenomenon has been variously identified as the apple, banana, and Oreo cookie syndrome (i.e., racially "red, yellow, or brown" on the outside and culturally "white" inside). Management of this problem is rarely simple. Adoptive parents can be threatened by their child's flight away from the family identity, while perhaps not understanding the depth of their adopted child's personal struggles (since they did not have a similar problem in their own youth). Conversely, the adoptee may be anguished at the biological parents' surrender of the child into the struggle alone. Obviously many cross-racial adoptees cope well with the situation, so such problems are not inevitable (Anthony and Cohler 1987). Should they occur, the psychiatrist must be adept at dealing with matters of racial, ethnic, and family identity, as well as self-identity

125

(Krener and Sabin 1985; Westermeyer 1979a, 1979c; Wolters 1980).

Unaccompanied refugee minors are also at risk to special management problems (Carlin 1986; Harding and Looney 1977; Looney 1979). Management depends not only upon a descriptive diagnosis, but also upon identifying pathogenic factors and dealing with them. Two or more pathogenic factors often coexist. Some of these may be ongoing and can interfere with current management. Common problems include the following:

- Placement in a culturally unfamiliar home, so that the minor has to acculturate in the absence of a culturally familiar family and an expatriate community (consider yourself being placed in a Cambodian family at age 14 or 15, and being unable to communicate with them);
- Loss of family members during refugee flight with the absence of a grieving period (and subsequent "missed grief" reactions);
- Preexisting psychopathology in the minor that led to the patient being sent away (e.g., mania, learning disorders, brain insult from trauma or malnutrition or infection, organic personality disorders, sociopathic personality);
- Psychopathology in the family of origin (e.g., schizophrenia, substance abuse, affective disorder), so that the minor is sent away or given up for adoption because the biological parent or parents cannot care for the child;
- Resentment at having to meet family expectations after living independently on the street or without parental supervision;
- Misunderstanding on the part of the minor, for example expecting that a welfare stipend belongs to the child exclusively;
- Unrealistic expectations by the family of origin that the unaccompanied minor will be economically successful in the new country and will be able to send money home to support the family;

- Family problems in the resettlement family that were either preexisting (i.e., the placement was sought in part to deal with dissension in the family) or precipitated by the mentally ill minor;
- Abuse of the unaccompanied minor in the resettlement home (e.g., physical abuse, sexual abuse, using the minor as an unpaid laborer);
- Social isolation of the minor away from other minors and adults of the same cultural group.

Acutely anxious, panicky, or severely anguished patients may leave assessment or early treatment if some level of relief is not immediately forthcoming. Although this can occur among native-born patients, it appears to be more likely among migrant patients. This flight from care may be due to the prevalence of anxiety disorders and agitated depression in this group, the tradition of seeking help from numerous healers in direct proportion to the perceived discomfort of the symptoms, the insecurity of being in an unfamiliar environment, or the lack of familiarity with psychiatric methods. Whatever the explanation, the psychiatrist should consider methods that can reduce the more acute and severe symptoms (e.g., nonsedative medication, relaxation techniques, milieu change, behavior modification). Probably more so than in native-born patients, migrant patients are apt to receive combined biomedical, psychotherapeutic, and sociotherapeutic modalities in the course of their care. Patients usually accept this multimodality approach well, but it can add to the clinical management burdens as well as to the cost and intensity of care, at least in the early phases of care.

Another cause for flight from care is the recurrent nature of certain psychiatric disorders among migrants. Posttraumatic stress disorders, major depressions, paranoid conditions, and acute psychoses often recur among migrants as they are reexposed to environmental stresses and losses (Kinzie and Fleck 1987). If the patient is alerted to the possibility of a recurrence, they are more apt to return in a timely fashion at the first indications of renewed symptoms. Current life events may precipitate posttraumatic stress disorder in victims of war and persecution even four or five decades after the original events (Krell 1988). In the case of certain recurrent problems, such as recurrent adjustment disorders or depression, the possibility of a personality disorder should be considered (Pilkonis and Frank 1988).

Psychiatric casualties returning home from other states or from abroad present a different group of management problems. Usually they have been hospitalized recently, are on medications, and are returning with a clinician or family member. They may require immediate hospitalization in order to continue their care. Even if immediate hospitalization has not been recommended by those transferring the patient, it may become necessary if the patient has difficulty reentering the former social network and community. The initial challenge for the psychiatrist consists of assuming the care of a person in "midstream," that is, at some point after treatment has been initiated but before an adequate recovery. This midstream therapeutic challenge requires that extra time be spent going over the patient's records (which should have accompanied the patient, but sometimes do not), communicating with those who have provided care so far (if possible), and spending extra time getting to know this partially treated patient.

Special Aspects of Management

Finances can obstruct proper psychiatric care of migrants, even though the professional and technical aspects of care might be excellent. Migrants who do not have access to health insurance or are not independently wealthy are vulnerable. They include many foreign students, refugees, illegal migrant workers, and unemployed in-country migrants. As the money available for psychiatric services has dwindled in recent years, the situation has become a bitter one in the United States. (Elsewhere, many countries provide psychiatric services for migrants on a par with those of local citizens.) Withholding services from migrants due to financial-administrative considerations occurs regularly throughout the United States, as in these recent cases:

- A psychotically depressed refugee living in a nearby state did not receive care because (1) no cross-cultural services were available in her state, (2) her state would not authorize care outside of the state, and (3) an appropriate hospital in a nearby state would not permit nonemergency hospitalization for an out-of-state person in the absence of guaranteed funding.
- An acutely psychotic foreign student from a private, out-of-state, religion-affiliated school cannot receive psychiatric care because (1) she has no medical insurance, (2) the school that accepted her has no provision for providing psychiatric services for students, and (3) her family will not permit her embassy to be contacted to pay for the services for fear of economic and possibly political reprisals against other family members at home.
- An American Indian patient with substance abuse, major depression, and HIV-positive serology cannot be accepted into a hospital day program because (1) he is from another state, so his care cannot be paid for locally, (2) his state has no program for HIV-positive substance abusers and yet will not pay for his care out of state, and (3) since he has not been living on a reservation and was not been referred from an Indian Health Service facility, the Bureau of Indian Affairs will not pay for his care.

Even when private insurance is available, the fee schedule does not take into account the special needs of some migrant patients. These special needs often lead to higher costs for care due to the following factors:

- Translators, interpreters, or bilingual psychiatric assistants must be recompensed for their time;

- Translation doubles the time required for communication;
- Extra time must be spent in understanding the patient's cultural background and stage of acculturation; at times this requires extra time with "cultural consultants" who must also be paid;
- Long-distance phone calls and letters are frequently needed to obtain an adequate premorbid history and history of previous psychiatric care;
- Education of the migrant patient is more time consuming on average than is education of the usual nonmigrant patient (e.g., regarding nature of the disorder, its causes, treatment, and prognosis);
- If the patient has not previously acculturated to the new society, and is not returning home, extra treatment time and rehabilitation services are needed to facilitate recovery and to prevent recurrence;
- For patients returning home, extra time is required for those initiating the transfer, implementing it, and accepting it on the receiving end.

Since fee-for-service programs contain these limitations for migrants, it had been anticipated that prepaid or health maintenance organizations (HMOs) would correct these inequities. Instead, they have often contributed to the problem by withholding timely and appropriate care.

Care in the public sector also can be problematic for migrants. Since many community mental health clinics are overworked and underfunded, their administrators and clinicians may shy away from any new group of patients—particularly patients who would require extra time, expertise, and staff to treat. Due to the absence of readily available outpatient services, such patients are apt to end up hospitalized in state hospitals. Lack of expert staff in state facilities may result in misdiagnosis and inappropriate care. States differ widely in the quality and availability of their public sector psychiatry, from fairly good to very poor and getting worse. Problems in the public sector relevant to migrants include the following: low levels of professional expertise for cross-cultural care and other migrant problems; low accessibility of services; poor continuity between inpatient and outpatient services; and jurisdictional problems, so that patients from other states and other countries are not readily served.

Illegal or "undocumented" migrants may avoid psychiatric care because this may result in their repatriation to the country of origin. Or in some states or communities, they may seek care but are refused it because they do not meet residency or citizenship requirements. For some, the alternative is deterioration, starvation, exposure, or violent death in the streets. Health care workers are left unsupported to manage such situations when border security is inadequate and local economic forces drive the use of cheap "wetback" labor. Such problems cannot be humanely and efficiently addressed by clinicians alone but need government and community involvement (Arnold 1979).

Legal and political problems may also intrude in the management of migrant patients. For example, courts conducting commitment proceedings are reluctant to commit persons from elsewhere if the local government has to bear the cost of psychiatric care. This results in migrants being released when, by local standards, they might otherwise be committed to treatment.

Concurrent folk therapies and religious rituals need not complicate treatment, especially when they are supportive in nature and, if taken internally, have mostly nutritional rather than neurotransmitter effects (Chak et al. 1984). Examples include the Last Rites of the Catholic Church, Midiwinin animistic healing rituals of the Chippewa people, or various soups or foods for certain symptoms. As familiar rituals in a time of crisis, these may aid in calming the patient, reassuring the patient and family that everything possible is being done, and affirming the concern and involvement of the patient's family and community (Atkinson 1987). Some therapies and rituals can seriously interfere with assessment, treatment, and recovery, however, as in these examples:

- Giving the patient or family to understand that failure to respond immediately is evidence of the patient's unworthiness or lack of faith;
- Insisting that the patient discontinue psychiatric care in order to obtain the other therapy or ritual;
- Requiring risky behaviors on the part of the patient (e.g., prolonged fasting, travel to a distant shrine);
- Application of over-the-counter or herbal caustic or potentially allergenic substances (with possible burns, gastric ulceration, corneal ulcerations, allergic dermatitis) (Foster and Sommer 1987; Perrault et al. 1988);
- Ingestion of herbal substances that can exacerbate psychiatric conditions or produce new psychiatric disorders (e.g., anticholinergic herbs, cannabis preparations, opium);
- Expenditures of large sums of family money to bring in healers or shamans from distant areas (e.g., from distant states, and even foreign countries).

In order to work with patients and families concurrently using other health care approaches, it is important to understand the methods and rationales of these other systems (Guilmet and Whited 1987). It then may be feasible to help the patient in benefiting from several systems at the same time, rather than forcing the patient to choose between them (Lee 1986).

Somatization can impede clinical management if the clinician permits the dialogue to remain on somatic topics alone. After somatic signs and symptoms have been explored thoroughly, it is important to move on to exploring psychophysiological symptoms (e.g., sleep disturbance, anorexia, anergy), emotional symptoms (e.g., crying spells, fears), mental symptoms (e.g., poor memory, trouble concentrating), interpersonal symptoms (e.g., social withdrawal, irritability), behavioral symptoms (e.g., agitation, self-destructive behavior), and Mental Status Examination (e.g., recall, cognition). Once rapport has been established and the presence of these symptoms has been identified, it is then possible to focus the interview on psychosocial issues. Most migrant patients presenting with somatization do not have somatoform disorder. In a series of 300 refugee patients at our facility, only 3 (1%) were diagnosed as having somatoform disorder whereas 49% had an affective disorder, 29% had an anxiety disorder, and 21% had various other disorders (e.g., organic brain syndrome, mental retardation). This trend for migrants to overemphasize somatic symptoms while underemphasizing psychosocial concerns has been observed in community surveys as well as in clinical studies (Young et al. 1987).

References

Anthony EJ, Cohler BJ: The Invulnerable Child. New York, Guilford, 1987

Arnold F: Providing medical services to undocumented immigrants: costs and public policy. International Migration Review 13:706–715, 1979

Atkinson JM: The effectiveness of shamans in an Indonesian ritual. American Anthropologist 89:342–355, 1987

Bernal Y Del Rio V: Psychiatric ethics and confidentiality, in Comprehensive Textbook of Psychiatry. Edited by Kaplan HI, Sadock BJ. Baltimore, Williams & Wilkins, 1985, pp 1998–2006

Carlin JE: Child and adolescent refugees: psychiatric assessment and treatment, in Refugee Mental Health in Resettlement Countries. Edited by Williams C, Westermeyer J. Washington, DC, Hemisphere, 1986, pp 131–140

Chak S, Nixon J, Dugdale A: Primary health care for Indo-Chinese children in Australia. Aust Paediatr J 20:57–58, 1984

Clement DC: Samoan folk knowledge of mental disorder, in Cultural Conceptions of Mental Health and Therapy. Edited by Marsella AJ, White GM. Boston, Reidel, 1982, pp 193–213

D'Andre R, Egan M: The colors of emotion. American Ethnologist 1:49–63, 1974

Deinard AS, Dunnigan T: Hmong health care—reflections on a six-year experience. International Migration Review 21:857–865, 1987

Dunnigan T: Segmentary kinship in an urban society: the Hmong of St. Paul-Minneapolis. Anthropological Quarterly 55:126–134, 1982

Edgerton RB: Conceptions of psychosis in four East African societies. American Anthropologist 68:408–425, 1966

Fabrega H, Metzger D: Psychiatric illness in a small Ladino community. Psychiatry 31:339–351, 1968

Foster A, Sommer A: Corneal ulceration, measles, and childhood blindness in Tanzania. Br J Ophthalmol 71:331–343, 1987

Guilmet GM, Whited DL: Cultural lessons for clinical mental health practice in the Puyallup tribal community. American Indian and Alaska Native Mental Health Research 1:32–49, 1987

Harding RK, Looney JG: Problems of Southeast Asian children in a refugee camp. Am J Psychiatry 134:407–411, 1977

Hoang GN, Erickson RV: Cultural barriers to effective medical care among Indochinese patients. Annu Rev Med 36:229–239, 1985

Jones IH, de la Horne DJ: Psychiatric disorders among Aborigines of the Australian western desert. Soc Sci Med 7:219–228, 1973

Kemp S, Williams K: Demonic possession and mental disorder in medieval and early modern Europe. Psychol Med 17:21–29, 1987

Kinzie JD: Cultural aspects of psychiatric treatment with Indochinese refugees. American Journal of Social Psychiatry 1:47–53, 1985

Kinzie JD, Fleck J: Psychotherapy with severely traumatized refugees. Am J Psychother 41:82–94, 1987

Krell R: Survivors of childhood experiences in Japanese concentration camps. Am J Psychiatry 145:383–384, 1988

Krener PG, Sabin C: Indochinese immigrant children: problems in psychiatric diagnosis. J Am Acad Child Psychiatry 24:453–458, 1985

Kroll J, Bachrach B: Medieval visions and contemporary hallucinations. Psychol Med 12:709–721, 1982

Lee PA: Traditional medicine: dilemmas in nursing practice. Nursing Administration Quarterly 10:14–20, 1986

Leighton AH, Lambo TA, Hughes CC, et al: Psychiatric Disorder Among the Yoniba. New York, Cornell University Press, 1963

Looney JG: Adolescents as refugees. Adolesc Psychiatry 7:199–208, 1979

Marsella AJ, White GM (eds): Cultural Conceptions of Mental Health and Therapy. Boston, Reidel, 1982

Masters R, Friedman LN, Getzel G: Helping families of homicide victims: a multidimensional approach. Journal of Traumatic Stress 1:109–125, 1988

Miller JG: Attitudes and social cognition: culture and the development of everyday social explanation. J Pers Soc Psychol 46:961–978, 1984

Muecke MA: Caring for Southeast Asian refugee patients in the USA. Am J Public Health 73:431–438, 1983

Murphy JM: Psychiatric labeling in cross cultural perspective. Science 191:1019–1028, 1976

Perrault J, Fleming R, Dozois RR: Surreptitious use of salicylates: a cause of chronic recurrent gastroduodenal ulcers. Mayo Clin Proc 63:337–342, 1988

Pilkonis PA, Frank E: Personality pathology in recurrent depression: nature, prevalence and relationship to treatment response. Am J Psychiatry 145:435–441, 1988

Resner R, Hartog J: Concepts and terminology of mental disorder among Malays. Journal of Cross Cultural Psychology 1:369–381, 1970

Roth S, Lebowitz L: The experience of sexual trauma. Journal of Traumatic Stress 1:79–107, 1988

Sokoloff B, Carlin J, Pham H: Five-year follow-up of Vietnamese refugee children in the United States. Clin Pediatr 23:565–570, 1984

Wallace AFC: Cultural determinants of response to hallucinatory experience. Arch Gen Psychiatry 1:58–69, 1959

Ward C, Beaubrun MH: Spirit possession and neuroticism in a West Indian Pentecostal community. Br J Clin Psychol 20:295–296, 1981

Westermeyer J: Ethnic identity problems among 10 Indian psychiatric patients. Int J Soc Psychiatry 25:188–197, 1979a

Westermeyer J: Folk concepts of mental disorder among the Lao: continuities with similar concepts in other cultures and in psychiatry. Culture, Medicine and Psychiatry 3:301–317, 1979b

Westermeyer J: The "apple" syndrome: the effects of racial-ethnic discontinuity. Journal of Operational Psychiatry 10:134–140, 1979c

Westermeyer J, Wintrob R: "Folk" criteria for the diagnosis of mental illness in rural Laos: on being insane in sane places. Am J Psychiatry 136:755–761, 1979a

Westermeyer J, Wintrob R: "Folk" explanations of mental illness in rural Laos. Am J Psychiatry 136:901–905, 1979b

White GM: Conceptual universals in interpersonal language. American Anthropologist 82:759–781, 1980

White GM, Marsella AJ: Introduction: cultural conceptions in mental health research and practice, in Cultural Conceptions of Mental Health and Therapy. Edited by Marsella AJ, White GM. Boston, Reidel, 1982 pp 1–38

Wolters WHG: Psychosocial problems in young foreign adopted children. Acta Paedopsychiatrica 46:67–81, 1980

Young RF, Bukoff A, Waller JB, Blount SB: Health status, health problems and practices among refugees from the Middle East, Eastern Europe and Southeast Asia. International Migration Review 21:760–782, 1987

Chapter 6
Somatotherapies

Chapter 6
Somatotherapies

Psychiatric care for migrants often involves the application of pharmacotherapies and other somatotherapies across a range of races and ethnicities. This process can require special knowledge and skills based on biological, psychological, or sociocultural differences among peoples. This chapter aims at alerting the clinician to potential differences, to the research indicating areas of similarities and differences, and to clinical methods that can be employed for maximal therapeutic benefit.

Factors Affecting Somatotherapies

Pharmacokinetics may vary across races and cultures (Kalow 1982). That is, a drug may be absorbed, distributed through the body, localized in tissues, metabolized, and excreted differently among various groups. For example, heavy tobacco smokers have been shown to require higher doses of neuroleptics and tricyclics, probably due to the enhanced activity of hepatic enzymes induced by chronic tobacco use (Linnoila et al. 1981). Similarly, depressed alcoholics and depressed patients who use alcohol have been observed to require higher doses of tricyclic medication (Ciraulo et al. 1982; Linnoila et al. 1981). Exposure to various chemicals can accelerate the elimination of tricyclics (Risch et al. 1981). Diet containing more protein can accelerate the metabolic rate of certain drugs, presumably by affecting protein binding in plasma (Branch et al. 1978; Kalow 1982). This is an important consideration, since 80–90% of most psychotropic agents are protein-bound in the bloodstream, and it is the nonbound portion of the drug that exerts its pharmacological effect (Forsman and Larsson 1978; Forsman and Ohman 1977). Race may affect protein binding. For example, Orientals and Occidentals have shown a difference in the protein binding of diphenhydramine, often used in conjunction with neuroleptics (Spector et al. 1980). Height, weight, differences in gastric acidity, and percent body fat—all potentially related to race and culture—can also affect the pharmacokinetics of drugs. Additional factors theoretically operating on pharmacokinetics might include food additives, use of over-the-counter (OTC) and herbal medications, and air pollution.

Pharmacodynamics refers to the neurotransmitter, neurophysiological, behavioral, psychological, and social effects of psychotropic drugs, along with their mechanisms of action (Melmon and Morelli 1978). A well-known example with alcohol is the flushing response, which has a variable distribution across races due to differences in enzymes acting on alcohol metabolism (Agarwal and Goedde 1986; Wolff 1972). Therapeutic response levels may also differ among cultural and ethnic groups. For example, in Japan the therapeutic blood lithium range for manic depressive patients and blood imipramine levels for depressed patients have been almost half of those observed in the West, and even in some parts of Asia (Okuma 1981; Takahashi 1979; Yamashita and Asano 1979). Although the mechanics of alcohol flushing have been well described, the relationships between differences in blood levels, therapeutic responses, and dosage are not so well understood. Possible explanations of differences include but are not limited to the following factors (Chrusciel 1978; Honda and Suzuki 1979; Korpi et al. 1983; Rawkins 1974; Shen and Zhang 1982):

- Pharmacokinetic factors (e.g., enzymatic differences);
- Pharmacodynamic factors (e.g., variable effects of medication on neurotransmitter systems);
- Social psychological differences (e.g., variation in tolerance to symptoms across cultures);
- Differences in clinical practice (e.g., physicians in diverse countries may practice more or less aggressive pharmacotherapy, or have differing access to modern monitoring methods such as blood levels);

- Sampling problems (e.g., patients versus normal subjects; or patients of differing severity may be compared with each other—a problem remedied in part by rating scales and other means of careful case description);
- Methodological problems (e.g., differences in laboratory methods and norms, compliance, time of dose, single versus repeated doses).

Traditional practices in folk pharmacotherapy can affect compliance with pharmacotherapy regimens (Opako 1986). Migrants from developing regions often possess an aspirin, penicillin, or herbal medicine approach to conceptualizing pharmacotherapy (Finkler 1985; Westermeyer 1983, 1988). That is, they expect rapid relief, perhaps within a few hours (e.g., aspirin for pain relief), or at least several days (e.g., penicillin for infection). If relief is not rapidly forthcoming, they may discontinue the medication or request a new one, or both (e.g., common herbal medicine practice). Typically also, these familiar pharmacotherapies involve few or no side effects. The dosages and duration of these medications are usually quite standard, so that the patients know the regimen from the beginning. Little or no change in the individual, the family, or other social units is required. Against these folk expectations, the use of psychotropic medications to treat psychiatric disorder is unfamiliar because these drugs typically involve the following:

- Gradual, sometimes almost imperceptible improvement over a period of weeks, with some residual symptoms that may not clear completely for several months to a few years;
- Notable side effects with some drugs in the therapeutic range (e.g., dry mouth and constipation with tricyclics, tremor or hypotension with neuroleptics, hypotension or confusion with high doses of blocking agents);
- Education regarding potential major complications of certain drugs [e.g., hypertension with monoamine oxidase (MAO) inhibitors, cardiac arrhythmias with tricyclics, priapism with

141

trazodone, tardive dyskinesia with neuroleptics, potential addiction with benzodiazepines];
- Dosage must be individualized, requiring more visits and time with the prescribing physician and at times involving repeated, expensive blood level monitoring (e.g., lithium, tricyclics);
- A variable duration of treatment, again with greater physician and medication expense due to prolonged, recurrent, or chronic nature of some psychiatric illness;
- Collateral or phased administration of medications, psychotherapies, and sociotherapies in many cases, so that one medication or even one modality may not be sufficient for a full course of treatment.

Specific inquiry should be made about use of folk remedies and OTC drugs from the migrant patient. Examples of folk remedies that affect response to psychiatric pharmacotherapies, as well as psychiatric status more generally, include the following:

- Phenacetin, acetominophen, or salicylates, either used surreptitiously in high doses for an "aspirin jag" or relief of tension, or used unknowingly in a folk nostrum by middleclass white Americans (Perrault et al. 1988);
- Various earths and clays, some of which may have pharmaceutical properties, by Afro-Americans and Asian immigrants (Vermeer and Farrell 1985);
- Herbal compounds containing cytotoxic substances, such as pennyroyal oil (Sullivan et al. 1979) or poke root (Lewis and Smith 1979) among rural or "anti-establishment" American herbalists;
- Warfarin-containing tonka beans, melilot, or woodruff among American herbalists (Hogan 1983);
- Toxic doses of licit substances, such as tobacco or coffee, administered by enema among American herbalists (Eisele and Reay 1980);
- Use of herbal emetics, antagonist drugs, or sweat baths, with

possible dehydration or electrolyte imbalance (Trotter 1979;
Westermeyer 1979);
- Arsenic or lead in folk preparations, especially used by Asian
  and Latin American immigrants (Kerr and Saryan 1986; Levitt
  1983; Sankury 1983; Trotter et al. 1983);
- Opium-containing folk compounds used by Hmong and other
  Indochinese refugees (Beraut and Lanzkowsky 1983; Wester-
  meyer 1983);
- Carcinogenic agents, such as comfrey root or tea used by
  American herbalists (Ames et al. 1987).

Folk somatotherapies besides pharmacotherapies can also
affect the clinical picture. For example, procedures that break
the skin with shared instruments expose the migrant patient
to possible blood-borne infections, such as hepatitis B or acquired immune deficiency syndrome (AIDS). This may occur
via contaminated acupuncture needles, healing or ritual tat-
toos, or needles (used by folk injectionists, who administer
self-prescribed medications on the streets in many developing
countries). Several folk therapies can produce hemorrhage or
tissue damage, including pinching, "coining" (abrading the skin
with the edge of a coin), deep vigorous massage, pounding
or beating, and scarification. These methods can produce an
abnormal dexamethasone suppression test (DST) or elevated
white blood count.

A key factor affecting decisions on somatotherapy is diagnosis. In order to benefit from research advances, clinicians
make accurate diagnoses using modern criteria (American Psychiatric Association 1980). Assessment of the migrant patient
is thus the first and most critical step in selecting and recommending treatment.

Pharmacotherapies

Tricyclic medications are commonly prescribed to migrant patients, given their high rates of Axis I DSM-III-R disorders,

including major depression, panic and other severe anxiety disorders, and depression associated with other disorders (e.g., shared delusional disorder, organic affective disorder). In light of the low tolerance of many migrant patients to side effects, tricyclics with low antihistaminic and anticholinergic side effects should be considered. Since migrants often have limited financial resources, compliance may be improved by prescribing the older and less expensive compounds. A drug such as imipramine comprises an adequate compromise. With outpatients, an effective strategy is to begin with a dose as small as 25 mg, adding 25 mg every day or two until side effects or therapeutic response is reached. Blood levels in 3 or 4 weeks help to assess dosage and to ascertain compliance. Somatizing patients appear to be at particular risk for noncompliance.

Intragroup variation in tricyclic pharmacokinetics greatly exceeds the observed intergroup differences (Potter et al. 1984; Sjoqvist and Bertilsson 1986; Yamashita and Asano 1979). However, pharmacokinetic studies on tricyclics have generally (but not always) shown some racial-ethnic differences. Several investigators have demonstrated that, when compared to Asians in the United States and the United Kingdom, Caucasians attained peak plasma levels later (Rudorfer et al. 1984) and had lower plasma levels over time (Allen et al. 1977; Lewis et al. 1980).

This difference appears to be due to a greater incidence of slow hydroxylation among Asians, compared to Caucasians (Inaba et al. 1981; Kalow 1982; Potter et al. 1984). Compared to black American patients, Caucasian Americans also showed lower plasma levels of tricyclics (Ziegler and Biggs 1977). On the other hand, Gaviria et al. (1986) failed to demonstrate any kinetic differences between Mexican-born and Anglo normals in the United States, using nortriptyline. Likewise, Pi et al. (1986) failed to show a difference in the plasma clearance of desipramine, comparing Asians and Caucasians. Overall, these data support the general clinical practice of careful individualization of tricyclic dosage—a procedure employed by most psychiatrists anyway.

Pharmacodynamic comparisons of tricyclics across ethnic groups are few in number. Marcos and Cancro (1982) reported that, compared to Anglo patients, depressed Puerto Rican patients reported twice as many side effects, yet required a lower dosage in order to attain therapeutic benefit. Despite these differences in dosage and side effects, similar proportions of patients recovered in both groups. Among depressed Colombian patients, Escobar and Tuason (1980) also found more side effects than among American patients, but—unlike Marcos and Cancro—they observed that a significantly higher percentage of Colombians improved on the medication. Sampling differences may have accounted for this finding. Ziegler and Biggs (1977) observed that, at a comparable dose, black patients manifested a more rapid clinical response and higher plasma levels compared with Caucasian patients. In line with these data, Livingston et al. (1983) noted that black patients may be at greater risk to confusion from tricyclics compared with Caucasian patients.

MAO inhibitors have not been carefully studied across groups. They do present particular problems in migrant patients apt to be taking OTC remedies containing sympathomimetic compounds and certain ethnic foods, especially aged sausages and aged fish sauce (Zisook 1985). In light of these risks and the likelihood of sympathomimetic exposure, some clinicians make a policy of not prescribing MAO inhibitors for migrants. This author has prescribed MAO inhibitors, but with extensive education and close monitoring (i.e., daily blood pressures as outpatients, or hospitalization for purposes of monitoring). Several migrant patients have had systolic blood pressure increases of 20–40 mmHg, and the MAO inhibitor has been discontinued. Predictably, a few more patients failed MAO inhibitor therapy after having failed tricyclic therapy; electroconvulsive therapy (ECT) eventually was effective. However, MAO inhibitors have been successfully used in several cases in which tricyclics were not desirable (e.g., abnormal ECGs) or had produced problematic side effects (e.g., hyperphagia and weight gain, severe constipation).

Lithium has proven effective among Japanese patients at blood levels well below those employed elsewhere, i.e., 0.4–0.8 mEq/L (Okuma 1981; Takahashi 1979). Taiwanese patients have been maintained at somewhat higher levels, around 0.5–0.8 mEq/L, with a mean of 0.71, but still lower than those in the United States (Chang et al. 1985; Yang 1985). Mean lithium levels in Shanghai, China, were 0.73 mEq/L as compared to 0.98 mEq/L among Caucasian patients in the United States (Chang et al. 1985). Despite these notable differences in prescribing practices, blood lithium levels among the Shanghai Chinese and American Caucasians were proportional to dosage, suggesting that there were no pharmacokinetic differences.

Racial differences in red blood cell (RBC) sodium and lithium levels have been recognized for some time. Trevisan et al. (1984) have studied the pharmacodynamic differences among black and white normal subjects in the United States, sampling in schools and places of employment. They found that whites of both sexes had higher sodium-lithium countertransport than blacks, but blacks had higher RBC sodium concentration than whites. This ambiguous finding is not consistent with the predicted direct relationship between countertransport and RBC sodium concentration (since both of these vary directly with blood pressure).

At this point the data demonstrate lithium-prescribing differences across national boundaries but do not indicate whether or not pharmacodynamic differences might also exist across races. Pharmacokinetic differences may exist, but then precise nature and clinical import have not been defined. Prescribing practices across races and cultures apparently need not be modified, with the exception of careful education regarding toxicity, the need for obtaining certain blood levels, and strictures against sharing medication with others.

Neuroleptics are prescribed for several clinical diagnoses prevalent among migrants, i.e., schizophreniform psychosis, mania, paranoia, psychotic depression not responding to antidepressant measures alone, shared delusional disorder, drug-precipitated psychoses, and organic brain syndromes. Migrants must frequently be on neuroleptic medication longer than might otherwise be the case. This is probably due to the ongoing stressors associated with acculturation and other adaptations to the new society (e.g., language, employment, social network reconstruction). At the same time, the prevalence of reactive psychosis and "good prognosis schizophrenia" (World Health Organization 1978) indicates the need to consider time-limited, rather than lifelong, neuroleptic regimens.

Pharmacokinetic studies have shown cross-racial differences in neuroleptics, similar to those of the tricyclics. Lin and Poland (1984) administered haloperidol to normal Asian and Caucasian volunteers in the United States. The Asians had significantly higher serum levels and a more pronounced prolactin response, as compared to the Caucasians. In a comparison of schizophrenic patients in Peking, China, and Caucasians in the United States, Potkin et al. (1984) likewise observed higher serum levels of haloperidol in the Chinese, using a fixed dose per weight over 6 weeks. Black inpatients have also shown higher blood levels per milligram dose of chlorpromazine as compared to white inpatients in the United States (Young 1986).

Pharmacodynamic studies tend to further support the pharmacokinetic findings. Two groups of investigators in California have found Asian-American patients to respond with lower neuroleptic doses than do Caucasian-American patients who were matched for demographic and clinical variables (Lin and Finder 1983; Yamamoto et al. 1979). Studies have shown that patients from Asia and the Middle East improve at medication levels that are less than those of Europeans and Caucasian Americans (Lewis et al. 1980; Okuma 1981). A comparison of Europeans and Caucasian Americans indicates that Europeans receive lower neuroleptic dosages (Denber et al. 1962). One group of investigators in the United States has failed to replicate the finding of neuroleptic dose differences between

Asian and Caucasian patients (Sramek et al. 1986). One American study showed Asian patients to have more extrapyramidal symptoms (EPS) than black or Caucasian patients (Binder and Levy 1981), but a study of African patients (Odejide 1980) revealed an EPS prevalence similar to that observed elsewhere. These differences in rates of EPS and serum levels may have implications for tardive dyskinesia (Jeste et al. 1979). These pharmacodynamic findings suggest that in addition to pharmacokinetic differences, there may be prescribing, social psychological, or environmental differences involved. As with tricyclic medication, the need for individualization of dosage for all patients is paramount.

Benzodiazepines and other sedatives present problems in the care of migrants for several reasons. First, a modicum of anxiety early on can be associated with eventual adaptation, whereas those who are void of anxiety may not strive to adapt (Westermeyer et al. 1984). Second, benzodiazepines interfere with memory, especially delayed recall, so that migrants may have difficulty with language acquisition and other recall-related acculturation tasks (Scharf et al. 1988). Third, the sedatives can disinhibit the control against violence, contributing to family abuse—already a problem in many migrant groups. Fourth, anxiety among migrants is apt to persist for months and even years, rather than to clear within days or a few weeks as often occurs among nonmigrant patients in crisis. This puts the migrant patient at risk to benzodiazepine addiction.

One study of diazepam in the United States failed to show a difference in its agonist effects when given to Asians and Caucasians (Ghoneim et al. 1981). Despite lack of sedation differences, Asians cleared the drug more slowly and had higher serum levels. Both groups had identical proportions of serum bound diazepam.

Analgesics are frequently prescribed for migrants in medical clinics in association with their high rates of somatization. Iatrogenic opioid addiction thus occurs as a complication. Nonopiate analgesics, such as phenacetin, acetominophen, acetylsalicyclic acid, ibuprofen, and similar compounds, are also liable to abuse by migrants. These latter compounds can produce medical problems, such as gastritis, esophagitis, peptic ulcer, bone marrow suppression, hepatic and renal tubular necrosis, and (for phenacetin) methemoglobinemia or hemolytic anemia.

Migrants are apt to experience chronic anxiety conditions, posttraumatic stress disorder (PTSD), or somatization associated with psychiatric conditions. In light of these common complaints, and the dangers from sedatives and analgesics, various other compounds have been employed in the care of migrants. Careful clinical studies regarding their use in migrants are not yet available. However, anecdotal cases and extrapolation from studies among nonmigrants do indicate their potential utility. The calcium channel blocker verapamil has proven effective in reducing the frequency of panic attacks, compared to placebo (Klein and Uhde 1988). These agents have also been used for a variety of other psychiatric disorders apt to occur in migrants, including affective disorder, organic syndromes, and other treatment-resistant problems (Pollack et al. 1987). The autonomic blocking agents propranolol and clonidine have been prescribed for chronic PTSD in combat veterans (Kolb et al. 1984). The availability of 7-day clonidine "patches" may be useful in some patients, particularly if oral pharmacophobia or compliance is a problem. Other medications successfully used for panic, obsessive compulsive disorders, PTSD, and phobias have included tricyclics, MAO inhibitors, and lithium (Walker 1982). Carbamazepine, an anticonvulsant with lithium-like properties in some patients (Post 1988), can aid patients with recurrent or cyclic affective disorders and organic brain syndromes, such as torture victims or those with head injuries (Ballenger 1988). Occasional neuroleptic-resistant psychotic patients manifesting aggression and interpersonal problems also respond to carbamazepine (Neppe 1988). As Friedman (1988) has emphasized, PTSD patients rarely respond to pharmacotherapy alone, but can benefit from medication along with individual, behavioral, or group psychotherapy. The same is true for most cases of anxiety disorder among migrants.

Disulfiram can aid in the recovery of alcoholic veterans, refugees, and other migrants, when prescribed in association with other modalities. Close monitoring by a physician during the early months of abstinence is always indicated. Patients with organic impairment or associated psychopathology (e.g., depression, schizophrenia), or patients who are on other psychotropic medications (e.g., anticonvulsants, tricyclics, neuroleptics) are apt to become confused or experience exacerbation of their psychopathology on ordinary doses of disulfiram (i.e., 250–500 mg). Reduction in dosage to 125 mg, or even 62.5 mg can relieve this problem, while still leaving the acetaldehyde reaction intact (Knee and Razani 1974; Westermeyer 1986).

Methadone withdrawal regimens are occasionally needed for traveling heroin addicts, iatrogenic opioid addicts, and refugee opium smokers. Opium addicts in North America are mostly ethnic Hmong from northern Laos, but some addicts are also ethnic Lao, Tai Dam, Mien, Vietnamese, and Chinese. Unlike heroin addicts who can often be withdrawn over 5–10 days, strongly addicted opium addicts may require 2 or 3 weeks due to the prolonged excretion of numerous opiate subcompounds. Longer regimens, up to 1 or 2 months, may be needed for elderly, postoperative, or chronically ill patients. Initial 24-hour doses of methadone range from 20 to 120 mg, depending on the patient's habit and severity of withdrawal (Westermeyer 1986).

After the methadone withdrawal regimen, and a Narcan challenge, it is then possible to initiate the long-acting antagonist naltrexone. This is a desirable regimen when patients continue to be exposed to the heroin or opium (as migrants often are). Intensive outpatient care should continue for 6–12 months, followed by another year of support and monitoring. Many successfully treated refugee addicts prefer to remain on naltrexone for 2 or 3 years, due to the prominence of craving at times of acculturation stress, episodic acculturation failures, and high exposure to opioids in many migrant patients. Stimulants, such as methylphenidate, can aid in the treatment of refugee children with attention deficit disorder (ADD), whether due to trauma, malnutrition, or infection. In treatment-resistant depressed patients, especially those who show evidence of brain disorder, a brief course of methylphenidate (carefully monitored) may be effective either alone or with tricyclics (Kaufman et al. 1984). Careful monitoring of outpatients is necessary to prevent stimulant abuse (by patient or other family member) and to detect such complications as worsening confusion or paranoid symptoms.

Other Somatotherapies

ECT has essentially the same indications for migrants as for nonmigrants, albeit with certain special considerations. Refugees and other migrants who present with psychotic conditions that have been present for many months or years may not respond to medications alone. After years of psychosis, with advanced deterioration, it may not be feasible to ascertain the diagnosis as precisely as with the usual patient. It is possible to achieve excellent results from ECT even in some deteriorated cases.

Fear of ECT occurs commonly among refugees, prisoners of war, victims of persecution and terror, and political exiles. Those who have been exposed to physical mistreatment by electricity, or by induced unconsciousness (by beating or inundation of the head, or asphyxiation) are apt to transfer these feelings to ECT. Rapport and trust in the physician, together with failed attempts at other treatment methods, are key elements in overcoming this fear. Meetings can be arranged between patients and families considering ECT and patients who have had ECT (along with the recovered patient's family). These meetings can be effective in reducing the extreme fear of ECT in some migrants.

Electrosleep or electroacupuncture consists of passing low voltage (around 9 to 12 volts) across the head, with electrodes or saline pads placed in the frontal or fronto-temporal regions, or with acupuncture needles placed in the ears. The method was developed before World War II by the Soviets, who found that this treatment temporarily relieved anxiety, agitation, anguish, chronic pain, and insomnia. During the period of Soviet-Chinese entente in the 1950s and 1960s, the Soviet electrosleep technology was integrated with Chinese acupuncture therapy, leading to electroacupuncture. The latter theory holds that the placement of the needles in specific "acupuncture meridians" is crucial, but the same result occurs whether or not precise meridians are employed (i.e., needles can be placed in the less painful lobe rather than in the more painful and infection-prone cartilaginous pinna). Either electrosleep or electroacupuncture can be useful in cases of acute adjustment syndromes, anxiety-related psychosomatic diseases, and drug withdrawal (Wen 1977; Wen and Chau 1973). With major or chronic disorders, however, these methods by themselves do not reverse basic psychopathological processes or enhance psychosocial adjustment (Whitehead 1978). Moreover, they can become used habitually by patients, leading to high treatment costs and to psychological "treatment dependency." This issue is especially relevant to migrants, who are apt to have major and/or chronic psychiatric disorders as well as somatization (i.e., somatic presentations of their psychosocial problems). Such patients are apt to become "treatment dependent" in association with acculturation failure and unemployment. Thus, it behooves programs offering these symptom-relieving modalities to employ them propitiously, carefully, and knowledgeably.

A 42-year-old Vietnamese refugee was seen on an emergency basis for urgent suicidal impulses. He was found to have severe melancholic depression, with a 20-lb weight loss, inability to work for several months, early morning wakening, feelings of hopelessness and worthlessness, and a plan to commit suicide. Over the previous year the patient had received weekly to twice-weekly electroacupuncture at a university-supported medical clinic that employed a Chinese acupuncturist. Indications for the acupuncture included back pain and headache along with anergy, fatigue, anorexia, and insomnia—i.e., depressive symptoms with presenting somatization. The patient responded to hospitalization and a course of tricyclic medication (250 mg imipramine were required to achieve therapeutic blood levels).

Acupuncture may appeal to planners because it is an apparently cost-effective approach. However, in the long run, it is not cost-effective if it relieves symptoms but does not reverse the progressive underlying disorder. Electrosleep or electroacupuncture may be employed for symptom relief in the early phases of psychiatric care for depressed or anxious patients with somatization, although one can also readily manage most of these patients without electrorelaxation methods.

Certain other problems attend the use of electroacupuncture. First, these treatments are expensive: a single treatment costs about the same as a brief visit with a psychiatrist, a 1-hour psychotherapy session with a social worker, or a few hours in an evening or day program. Second, the therapeutic use of needles in the clinic promulgates the folk therapy use of needles in the migrant community, fostering the spread of hepatitis B and other blood-borne infections. Third, it reinforces the somatizer's false notion that the cause of the symptoms is exclusively in the body rather than also in the patient's mind, life, and environment. This can dissuade patients from finding ways to deal more effectively with their lives. Fourth, the short-term efficacy of electrorelaxation (like that of benzodiazepines and other sedatives) can tend to undermine the mild to moderate anxiety that migrants must tolerate and use in order to facilitate their adjustments in the new environment.

Restraints are seldom necessary for violent migrants, as with patients in general; but they are sometimes necessary to protect the patient or others. Restraints are well known even as a folk method of containing dangerous behavior (Westermeyer and Kroll 1978). Crisis intervention, intensive nursing care, alleviation of stressful situations, resolution of intoxicated states, or medication in adequate doses can diminish the duration of restraints. Likewise, hospitalization on a locked unit or brief periods of seclusion can also prove effective, as with other patients.

A 20-year-old vacationer had been using amphetamines in order to study for final exams, before embarking on a month-long excursion with three classmates. During the trip she began smoking cannabis several times a day. One week into the vacation she began hearing voices and developed the delusion that she could kill people with her eyes. In order to avert this delusional consequence, she slashed her right eye with a razor blade and was restrained by her friends as she attempted to slash the other. Hospitalized on a surgical ward for care of her severely damaged eye (which required enucleation), she was not restrained and was allowed to smoke. She next proceeded to burn the cornea of her remaining eye with a cigarette. Transferred to a psychiatric unit, restraints were then applied and she was begun on a course of ECT. The patient made a full recovery of her drug precipitated psychosis and her episodic drug abuse. Following care for the injured cornea in her remaining eye, she was subsequently able to return to college, graduate, and enter her chosen profession.

Phototherapy can be important in selected cases of recurrent depression with a seasonal periodicity (Wehr et al. 1986, 1987). Many refugees, foreign students, and other immigrants in recent years have followed a tropical-to-temperate zone pathway. Consequently, winter-onset depression among migrants poses a common problem. Case reports suggest that other disorders may also be related to season, such as the premenstrual syndrome (Parry et al. 1987), overeating, and carbohydrate craving. Light exposure to the retina rather than to the skin may be the operant mechanism, although placebo responses have still not been fully assessed (Wehr et al. 1987). Seasonal following-the-sun migration may help some patients in using natural phototherapy to ameliorate their conditions.

154

A 43-year-old woman from South America had two decades of late-fall-onset depression since coming to the United States. Like many seasonal-onset depressed patients, she also had migraines, carbohydrate craving, overeating, and a family history of recurrent seasonal depression. During recurrences she required 200–350 mg imipramine plus thyroid to achieve therapeutic response. Return home to South America in the fall (when it is seasonally spring) modified her recurrent depressions. She was able to reduce her prophylactic imipramine dosage from 100–125 mg down to 25–50 mg.

Implementing the Somatotherapy Plan

Compliance problems can be a special problem for migrant patients who are unfamiliar with modern psychiatric pharmacotherapy (Meucke 1983). Those expecting rapid relief, little or no side effects, permanent medication-induced cures, and total relief from medication alone are highly apt not to comply, since their expectations diverge so greatly from the realities of care. Migrant patients likely to present compliance problems have one or more of the following characteristics: have limited education (or are illiterate); come from countries with limited medical services in which chronic disorders (e.g., hypertension) receive little attention; come from areas without psychiatric services; have been in the country for a brief period; if in the country a long time, have not acculturated and are culturally isolated; are mistrustful, or even suspicious of the health care system; are using their own folk resources that promise immediate relief via mechanistic interventions; do not understand the nature of the disorder or the rationale for the medical regimen; are unfamiliar regarding procedures for dealing with side effects or minor complications (such as calling the psychiatrist or going to the emergency department of the hospital); prematurely cease medication when target symptoms are much reduced or relieved; have complex or inconvenient drug regimes; or have had untoward experience with past prolonged regimens, such as prophylactic isoniazid hydrochloride (INH) for positive tuberculin tests (Meucke 1983).

Patient and family education is a key antidote to noncompliance. As in all education, one must start with the learner's knowledge base and build new information onto this existing infrastructure. This process calls for flexibility, as migrant patients range from illiterate to highly educated. Even among illiterate patients, one starts with some notions of health and disease, function and dysfunction that can be employed to the patient's benefit. All societies possess such concepts, which have been studied under the rubric *ethnopsychiatry*. Modal mental illness concepts present in many societies resemble the English folk terms *insanity* or *madness, nervous breakdown, mental retardation, character problem,* and *brain disease or damage* (Bhattacharyza 1986; Westermeyer 1981). Folk theories that can be employed as a conceptual infrastructure for pharmacotherapy include the following: humoral theories, including water, air, earth, blood, and bile (in parts of Southeast and South Asia, Middle East, Latin America); hot-cold foods, agents, or therapies (Latin America, Asia); yin-yang balances in the body (East Asia); life stresses, losses, or worries as causes for bodily imbalances (virtually universal); and childhood, constitutional, genetic, and family predispositions and vulnerabilities (virtually universal).

It is important, whenever possible, to become acquainted with such concepts prevalent in the patient's reference group. It is likewise critical not to apply group generalizations to individual patients and their families, but to discover their individual ideas about the clinical problem at hand. As has been noted in cross-cultural studies, cultural generalizations and the case-specific explanations do not always coincide (Westermeyer and Wintrob 1979a, 1979b).

Informed consent can present challenges in caring for migrant patients who, by virtue of limited literacy, education, or life experience, may not be able to appreciate the nuances of recommended treatments as fully as the average indigenous patient. An additional problem involves the related issues of likelihood of therapeutic benefit from the treatment (almost never 100%) and the risk of serious, potentially disabling or life-threatening complications (e.g., tardive dyskinesia from neuroleptics, cardiac complications of tricyclics, hypertension with MAO inhibitors). Traditional notions in many areas infer that recovery should be 100% (if patients believe in and comply with the treatment) and that treatment risks are small or nil (as is largely true of many placebo-like folk therapies). Scientific reality is obviously at odds with patient expectation in these regards. Many illiterate or poorly educated people, although perhaps intelligent and practical, have difficulties understanding probability and statistics—the bases of much modern clinical decision making. Clinicians who accurately describe the risks and complications of treatment in exquisite detail may be viewed as discouraging certain patients from treatment. The American legal concept of the "reasonable mind" (*mens rea*) often does not apply, if one applies modern American concepts. Clinicians must at times steer a tortuous course among such factors as the migrant patient's right to choose treatment, the patient's trust, the family's expectations, the clinical realities with and without treatment, and the forensic abstractions.

As indicated in the previous paragraph, the psychiatrist attending to migrant patients must make recommendations and commitments to treatment courses. At the same time, it is important to enhance patient decision making so as to enhance compliance. One important factor lies in the fact that, outside of Euroamerican value systems, the ideal locus of control often rests with the family or clan rather than with the individual. Thus, migrant families may be accustomed to making critical decisions regarding treatment, with limited input from the patient. Traditional family systems can greatly enhance patient compliance, so it is important to work with and within these systems. A proven modus operandi involves the following:

1. Convey the diagnosis and the recommended intervention to the patient and to the family unit;

2. Ensure that the family as well as the patient achieve optimal understanding of the diagnosis, the prognosis with and without treatment, and the advantages and liabilities associated with treatment;
3. Clarify expectations of the patient and family in the treatment process; and
4. Permit a period of hours or days for the patient and family to discuss and negotiate their willingness to accept and contribute to the treatment process.

Failure to take adequate time for decision making can result in serious miscommunication, with the patient and family appearing to respond positively in order to please the clinician, when in fact they have no intention of complying with the plan.

The involvement of a staff member from the same ethnic group as the patient can facilitate rapport, communication, trust, and commitment. Even if the psychiatrist has limited understanding of the patient's awareness of the problem, fellow expatriates can usually bridge these conceptual gaps.

Vehicles for administrating medication can be critical in compliance. As with most patients, the majority of migrant patients can take medication in pill form. At this point in world history, virtually all adult patients have taken pills in some form. Migrant children, adolescents, or elderly may have difficulty swallowing large tablets or capsules, so that a fluid vehicle is needed. Clinicians can mistakenly view migrant patients as naïve, trusting, or totally compliant, compared with their native-born patients. This erroneous viewpoint can easily evolve, since migrant patients often want to appear compliant or nonconfrontational in order to ensure help, even if they do not want to comply with certain aspects of care. Consequently, some migrant patients report taking medications at a prescribed level, when in fact they are not taking the medicine, "cheeking" them and spitting them out (if in the hospital), or taking them but at a reduced dosage. Methods of avoiding this problem can include liquid vehicles for hospitalized patients, or depot injections of neuroleptics. Topical patches (e.g., 7-day clonidine patches) are a familiar vehicle for many Asians accustomed to topical medication and application of bandages or topical salves to painful or symptomatic areas of the body.

Monitoring treatment, always important, assumes even greater significance with migrant patients, given the propensity for noncompliance. Without attention to monitoring, the psychiatrist may not accurately assess the causes for inadequate treatment response or treatment failure—a critical step in deciding on subsequent treatment steps. For example, a failure of outpatient tricyclic treatment for depression could imply that the next step should be either inpatient ECT, or an inpatient course of tricyclic therapy, or an outpatient trial of an MAO inhibitor, depending on the facts of the particular case. Monitoring should involve as many sources of data as possible, covering as many areas of treatment compliance and response as feasible. Examples include the following: the psychiatrist's own observations of the patient; the patient's self-report, including the internal consistency of these reports; observations and evaluations by other treating staff members; reports and opinions of patient's family, friends, and other collateral sources; clinical rating scales repeated over time [e.g., Hamilton scales for anxiety and depression, Brief Psychiatric Rating Scale (BPRS), Global Assessment Scale (GAS)]; self-rating scales repeated at intervals [e.g., 90-item Symptom Checklist (SCL-90), Zung or Beck depression scales]; laboratory reports, such as therapeutic blood levels [e.g., lithium (Prien 1979), neuroleptics (Shvartsburd et al. 1983), tricyclics (Risch et al. 1981)], or improving tests [e.g., dexamethasone suppression test (DST) for depression, gamma glutamyl transferase (GGT) for alcoholism] or toxic screens (e.g., cannabis or opiates in urine).

Phases of somatotherapy are largely similar among migrants and nonmigrants, with modifications in certain populations (e.g., those unfamiliar with psychiatric somatotherapies). These have been touched on elsewhere but are listed here to emphasize the changing therapeutic tasks for the psychiatrist over time. Special issues to be considered at each phase of care are as follows:

- Early: establishment of trust and rapport; education of patient and family regarding the disorder and recommended somatotherapy; treatment decision making; commitment of patient, family, and physician to the treatment course; initiation of therapy; and therapy management to achieve optimal dosage or intensity;
- Middle: assessing treatment (e.g., re-interviews, blood levels, nursing notes, family reports), heading off premature termination of therapy, possible addition of other therapies, and dealing with side effects or complications;
- Late: decreasing dosage or intensity of treatment, observing for recurrence of symptoms, following the patient beyond the cessation of somatotherapy, and assessing the need for other therapies (i.e., psychotherapies, somatotherapies).

Combining somatotherapies with other therapies (i.e., psychotherapies and sociotherapies), part and parcel of most psychiatrists' work, can present a few surprises in caring for migrant patients. These are largely covered in Chapters 7 and 8. Suffice it to say here that entree to remedial psychotherapies and sociotherapies must often begin with skillfully applied somatotherapies. These include such frequently encountered problems as psychotic depression, most melancholic depressions, long-standing major depression of simple type, paranoid psychoses, mania, certain organic and substance abuse disorders, and some severe anxiety disorders. A modicum of success in the somatotherapy arena can greatly foster compliance in other therapies, even among illiterate patients unable to speak the clinician's language and unfamiliar with other psychiatric modalities.

References

Agarwal DD, Goedde HW: Ethanol oxidation: ethnic variations in metabolism and response, in Ethnic Differences in Reactions to Drugs and Xenobiotics. Edited by Kalow W, Goedde HW, Agarwal DP. New York, Alan Liss, 1986, pp 99–112

Allen JJ, Rack PH, Vaddadi KS: Differences in the effects of clomipramine on English and Asian volunteers: preliminary report on a pilot study. Postgrad Med J 53:79–86, 1977

American Psychiatric Association: Diagnostic and Statistical Manual of Mental Disorders, Third Edition. Washington, DC, American Psychiatric Association, 1980

Ames BN, Magaw R, Gold LS: Ranking possible carcinogenic hazards. Science 236:271–280, 1987

Ballenger JC: The clinical use of carbamazepine in affective disorders. J Clin Psychiatry 49:13–19, 1988

Beraut M, Lanzkowsky P: Rare medical occurrences in Jewish traditions. JAMA 250:2469–2470, 1983

Bhattacharyza DP: Pagalami: Ethnopsychiatric Knowledge in Bengal. Syracuse, NY, Syracuse University Press, 1986

Binder R, Levy R: Extrapyramidal reactions in Asians (letter). Am J Psychiatry 138:1243–1244, 1981

Branch RA, Sahih SY, Momeida A: Racial differences in drug metabolizing ability: a study with antipyrine in the Indian. Clin Pharmacol Ther 24:283–286, 1978

Chang SS, Pandey GW, Yang YY, et al: Lithium pharmacokinetics: interracial comparison. Unpublished paper presented at annual meeting of the American Psychiatric Association, Dallas, TX, 1985

Chrusciel TL: Questions we recognize but cannot formulate. International Pharmacopsychiatry 13:112–117, 1978

Ciraulo DA, Anderson LM, Chapron DJ, et al: Imipramine deposition in alcoholics. J Clin Psychopharmacol 2:2–7, 1982

Denber HCB, Bente D, Rajotte P: Comparative analysis of the action of butyrylperazine at Manhattan State Hospital and the University Psychiatric Clinic at Erlangen. Am J Psychiatry 119:203–206, 1962

Eisele JW, Reay DT: Deaths related to coffee enemas. JAMA 244:1608–1609, 1980

Escobar JI, Tuason VB: Antidepressant agents—a cross-cultural study. Psychopharmacol Bull 16:49–52, 1980

Finkler K: Spiritualist Healers in Mexico: Success and Failures of Alternate Therapeutics. New York, Praeger, 1985

Forsman A, Larsson M: Metabolism of haloperidol. Current Therapeutic Research 24:567–569, 1978

Forsman A, Ohman R: Applied pharmacokinetics of haloperidol in man. Current Therapeutic Research 21:396–411, 1977

Friedman MJ: Toward rational pharmacotherapy for posttraumtic stress disorder: an interim report. Am J Psychiatry 1435:281–285, 1988

Gaviria M, Gill AA, Javaid JI: Nortriptyline kinetics in Hispanic and Anglo subjects. J Clin Psychopharmacol 6:227–231, 1986

Ghoneim MM, Korttila K, Chiang CK, et al: Diazepam effects and kinetics in Caucasians and Orientals. Clin Pharmacol Ther 19:749–756, 1981

Honda Y, Suzuki T: Transcultural pharmacokinetic study on Li concentration in plasma and saliva. Psychopharmacol Bull 15:37–39, 1979

Hogan RP: Hemorrhagic diathesis caused by drinking an herbal tea (letter). JAMA 249:2679, 1983

Inaba T, Otton S, Kalow W: Debrisoquine hydroxylation capacity: problems of assessment in two populations. Clin Pharmacol Ther 29:218–233, 1981

Jeste DV, Rosenblatt JE, Wagner RL, et al: High serum neuroleptic levels in tardive dyskinesia? (letter). N Engl J Med 301:1184, 1979

Kalow W: Ethnic differences in drug metabolism. Clin Pharmacokinet 7:373–400, 1982

Kaufman MW, Cassem NH, Murray GB: Use of psychostimulants in medically ill patients with neurological disease and major depression. Can J Psychiatry 29:46–49, 1984

Kerr HD, Saryan L: Arsenic content of homeopathic medicines. J Toxicol Clin Toxicol 24:451–459, 1986

Klein E, Uhde TW: Controlled study of verapamil for treatment of panic disorder. Am J Psychiatry 145:431–434, 1988

Knee ST, Razani J: Acute organic brain syndrome: complications of disulfiram therapy. Am J Psychiatry 131:1281–1282, 1974

Kolb LC, Burris BC, Griffiths S: Propranolol and clonidine in treatment of the chronic post-traumatic stress disorders of war, in Post-Traumatic Stress Disorder: Psychological and Biological Sequelae. Edited by van der Kolk BA. Washington, DC, American Psychiatric Press, 1984, pp 97–107

Korpi E, Phelps B, Granger H, et al: Simultaneous determination of haloperidol and its reduced metabolite in serum and plasma by isocratic liquid chromatography with electrochemical detection. Clin Chem 29:624–628, 1983

Levitt C: Folk remedy-associated lead poisoning in Hmong children. JAMA 250:3149–3150, 1983

Lewis P, Rack PH, Vaddadi KS, et al: Ethnic differences in drug response. Postgrad Med J 56 (suppl 1):46–49, 1980

Lewis WH, Smith PR: Poke root herbal tea poisoning. JAMA 242:2759–2760, 1979

Lin KM, Finder EJ: Neuroleptic dosage in Asians. Am J Psychiatry 140:490–491, 1983

Lin KM, Poland RE: Variation in neuroleptic response: Asians vs. Caucasians. Unpublished paper presented at annual meeting of Society for the Study of Culture and Psychiatry, Santa Fe, NM, 1984

Linnoila M, George L, Guthrie S, et al: Effect of alcohol consumption and cigarette smoking on antidepressant levels of depressed patients. Am J Psychiatry 138:841–842, 1981

Livingston RL, Zucker DK, Isenberg K, et al: Tricyclic antidepressants and delirium. J Clin Psychiatry 44:173–176, 1983

Marcos LR, Cancro R: Pharmacotherapy of Hispanic depressed patients: clinical observations. Am J Psychother 36:505–512, 1982

Melmon K, Morelli H: Clinical Pharmacology: Basic Principles in Therapeutics. New York, Macmillan, 1978, pp 951–981

Meucke MA: Caring for Southeast Asian refugee patients in the USA. Am J Public Health 73:431–438, 1983

Neppe VM: Carbamazepine in nonresponsive psychosis. J Clin Psychiatry 49:22–30, 1988

Odejide A: Prevalence of persistent abnormal involuntary movements among patients in a Nigerian long-stay psychiatric unit. International Pharmacopsychiatry 15:292–300, 1980

Okuma T: Differential sensitivity to the effects of psychotropic drugs: psychotics vs. normals; Asians vs. Western populations. Folia Psychiatrica et Neurologica Japonica 35:79–81, 1981

Opako DT: The impact of traditional African medicine on the use of modern drugs, in Ethnic Differences in Reactions to Drugs and Xenobiotics. Edited by Kalow W, Goedde HW, Agarwal DP. New York, Alan Liss, 1986, pp 59–75

Pantuck E, Panntuck C, Anderson K, et al: Cigarette smoking and chlorpromazine disposition and actions. Clin Pharmacol Ther 321:533–538, 1982

Parry BL, Rosenthal NE, Tamaskin L, et al: Treatment of a patient with seasonal premenstrual syndrome. Am J Psychiatry 144:762–766, 1987

Perrault J, Fleming CR, Dozois RR: Surreptitious use of salicylates: a cause of chronic recurrent gastroduodenal ulcers. Mayo Clin Proc 63:337–342, 1988

Pi E, Simpson G, Cooper T: Pharmacokinetics of desipramine in Caucasian and Asian volunteers. Am J Psychiatry 143:1174–1176, 1986

Pollack MH, Rosenbaum JF, Hyman SE: Calcium channel blockers in psychiatry. Psychosomatics 28:356–369, 1987

Post RM: Time course of clinical effects of carbamazepine: implications for mechanisms of action. J Clin Psychiatry 49 (suppl):35–48, 1988

Potkin SG, Shen Y, Pardes H, et al: Haloperidol concentrations elevated in Chinese patients. Psychiatry Res 12:167–172, 1984

Potter WZ, Rudorfer MV, Lane EA: Active metabolites of antidepressants: pharmacodynamics and relevant pharmacokinetics. Adv Biochem Psychopharmacol 39:373–390, 1984

Prien R: Discussion of lithium treatment in affective disorders: therapeutic plasma level (letter). Psychopharmacol Bull 15:35, 1979

Rawkins M: Variability in response to drugs. Br Med J 4:91–94, 1974

Risch SC, Kalin NH, Janowsky DS: Indications and guidelines for plasma tricyclic antidepressant concentration monitoring. J Clin Psychopharmacol 1:59–63, 1981

Rudorfer MV, Lan EA, Chang WH, et al: Desipramine pharmacokinetics in Chinese and Caucasian volunteers. Br J Clin Pharmacol 17:433–440, 1984

Sankury T: Lead poisoning from Mexican folk remedies—California (letter). JAMA 250:3149, 1983

Scharf MB, Fletcher K, Graham JP: Comparative amnestic effects of benzodiazepine hypnotic agents. J Clin Psychiatry 49:134–137, 1988

Shen Y, Zhang W: Psychiatric service in the People's Republic of China. Chin Med J 95:443–448, 1982

Shvartsburd A, Dekirmenjian H, Smith RC: Blood levels of haloperidol in schizophrenic patients. J Clin Psychopharmacol 3:7–12, 1983

Sjoqvist F. Bertilsson L: Slow hydroxylation of tricyclic antidepressants—relationship to polymorphic drug oxidation, in Ethnic Differences in Reactions to Drugs and Xenobiotics. Edited by Kalow W, Goedde HW, Agarwal DP. New York, Alan Liss, 1986, pp 169–188

Spector R, Choudhury A, Chiang C, et al: Diphenhydramine in Orientals and Caucasians. Clin Pharmacol Ther 28:229–234, 1980

Sramek J, Sayles M, Simpson G: Neuroleptic dosage for Asians: a failure to replicate. Am J Psychiatry 143:535–536, 1986

Sullivan JB, Rumack BH, Thomas H, et al: Pennyroyal oil poisoning and hepatotoxicity. JAMA 242:2873–2874, 1979

Takahashi R: Lithium treatment in affective disorders: therapeutic plasma level. Psychopharmacol Bull 15:32–35 1979

Trevisan M, Ostrow D, Cooper RS, et al: Sex and race differences in sodium-lithium countertransport and red cell sodium concentration. Am J Epidemiol 120:537–541, 1984

Trotter RT: Evidence of an ethnomedical form of aversion therapy on the United States-Mexico border. J Ethnopharmacol 1:279–284, 1979

Trotter RT, Ackerman A, Rodman D, et al: "Azarcon" and "Gaeta": ethnomedical solution to epidemiological mystery. Medical Anthropology Quarterly 14:3–18, 1983

Vermeer DE, Farrell RE: Nigerian geophagical clay: a traditional antidiarrheal pharmaceutical. Science 227:634–636, 1985

Walker JI: Chemotherapy of traumatic war stress. Milit Med 147:1029–1033, 1982

Wehr TA, Jacobsen FM, Sack DA, et al: Phototherapy of seasonal affective disorder. Arch Gen Psychiatry 43:870–874, 1986

Wehr TA, Skwerer RG, Jacobsen FM, et al: Eye versus skin phototherapy of seasonal affective disorder. Am J Psychiatry 144:753–761, 1987

Wen HL: Fast detoxification of drug abuse by acupuncture and electrical stimulation (A.E.S.) in combination with naloxone. Modern Medicine of Asia 13:13–17, 1977

Wen HL, Chau K: Status asthmaticus treated by acupuncture and electro stimulations. Asian Journal of Medicine 9:191–195, 1973

Westermeyer J: Medical and nonmedical treatment for narcotic addicts: a comparative study from Asia. J Nerv Ment Dis 167:205–211, 1979

Westermeyer J: Poppies, Pipes and People: Opium and Its Use in Laos. Berkeley, CA, University of California Press, 1983

Westermeyer J: A Clinical Guide to Alcohol and Drug Problems. New York, Praeger, 1986

Westermeyer J: Folk medicine in Laos: a comparison between two ethnic groups. Soc Sci Med 27:769–778, 1988

Westermeyer J, Kroll J: Violence and mental illness in a peasant society: characteristics of violent behavior and "folk" use of restraints. Br J Psychiatry 133:529–548, 1978

Westermeyer J, Wintrob R: "Folk" criteria for the diagnosis of mental illness in rural Laos. Am J Psychiatry 136:755–761, 1979a

Westermeyer J, Wintrob R: "Folk" explanations of mental illness in rural Laos. Am J Psychiatry 136:901–905, 1979b

Westermeyer J, Zimmerman R: Lao folk diagnoses for mental disorders: a comparison with psychiatric diagnoses. Med Anthropol 5:425–443, 1981

Westermeyer J, Vang TF, Neider J: Symptom change over time among Hmong refugees: psychiatric patients versus nonpatients. Psychopathology 17:168–177, 1984

Whitehead PC: Acupuncture in the treatment of addiction: a review and analysis. Int J Addict 13:1–16, 1978

Wolff P: Ethnic differences in alcohol sensitivity. Science 175:449–450, 1972

World Health Organization: The International Pilot Study of Schizophrenia, Vol II. Geneva, World Health Organization, 1978

Yamamoto J, Fung D, Lo S: Psychopharmacology for Asian Americans and Pacific Islanders. Psychopharmacol Bull 15:29–31, 1979

Yamashita I, Asano Y: Tricyclic antidepressants: therapeutic plasma level. Psychopharmacol Bull 15:40–41, 1979

Yang YY: Prophylactic efficacy of lithium and its effective

plasma levels in Chinese bipolar patients. Acta Psychiatr Scand 71:171–175, 1985

Young RC: Plasma nor$_1$-chlorpromazine concentrations: effects of age, race, and sex. Therapeutic Drug Monitoring 8:23–26, 1986

Ziegler VE, Biggs JT: Tricyclic plasma levels: effects of age, race, sex and smoking. JAMA 283:2167–2169, 1977

Zisook S: A clinical overview of monoamine oxidase inhibitors. Psychosomatics 26:240–251, 1985

Chapter 7
Psychotherapies

Chapter 7
Psychotherapies

Psychotherapy is sometimes viewed as a Western, solely American or European, and largely urban treatment modality that cannot be applied to non-Western, minority, or rural patients. This ethnocentric perspective fails to take into account the many common practices shared by healers through time and across cultures, including general medical practitioners, shamans, and even diviners and astrologers. Tseng and McDermott (1975) have listed these universal elements as follows:

1. Basic operations: identifying and naming the problem, prescribing a remedy, implementing treatment;
2. Elements of treatment: a period of orientation to the healing activity, establishing a therapist-patient relationship in which the presence of the therapist becomes a healing vehicle, establishing a culturally consistent context or "theater" for therapeusis (e.g., appropriate dress, behavior, certificate or license, office decor, institutional setting);
3. Defining the cause(s) of the problem: via dialogue, dreams, examination, psychometrics, laboratory tests, genetic maps;
4. Explaining the problem: patient comes to understand the problem in a way that is comprehensible and meaningful from the perspective of the patient's world view;
5. Prescription for change: change in patient's attitude or behavior, family change, healing ritual or ceremony, medication.

Despite these universal dimensions of therapy, all therapies and therapists are also culture-specific to some extent (Pedersen 1982). Therapist-patient differences in norms and values, culturally determined goals of therapy, cultural definitions of "reality" and "appropriate behavior," the relative weight accorded the individual versus the society, therapist prescriptions for "time out" from social roles and responsibilities and other ingrained facets of treatment exemplify the impossibility of a "culture-free" therapy. In fact, the culture-bound aspect of therapy is often a key feature in change and rehabilitation. Migrants can come to know and understand the new community and culture through therapy and through the indigenous therapist. To a certain extent, the patient's relationship with the therapist can become a microcosm for working out relationships with the new society. Acceptance of the therapist can symbolize acceptance by the receiving community. This can be a powerful factor in facilitating an "at home" feeling for the migrant patient. Even on a short-term basis, such a therapeutic relationship can be greatly comforting. For example, a psychiatrist visiting a remote area of Micronesia developed a painful and disabling musculotendinous problem and was treated by a local healer (using massage, manipulation, and reassurance). Another psychiatrist visiting a remote area of Southeast Asia developed a severe diarrhea and was treated with two pipes of opium, dietary recommendations, and reassurance. Both clinicians reported a remarkable immediate relief of their severe discomfiture and incapacitating symptoms, along with the ability to resume their travels. It seems likely that human succor by local people, for threatening symptoms in a remote and unfamiliar locale, was at least as powerful an antidote as the respective somatotherapies.

It should be kept in mind that psychotherapy may also have the potential for exacerbating the patient's condition. This may occur if the therapy undermines the patient's relationships with ethnic peers, or if it undermines coping behaviors that are adaptive in the patient's milieu. For example, excessive emphasis on individualism can cripple a patient who must adjust to a clan-centered society. Or guidance in dealing with a particular social problem in the United States could prove maladaptive, or even dangerous if attempted once the migrant returns to the home community.

Doctor-Patient Relationship

Mutual expectations between the psychiatrist and the migrant patient may differ, especially for patients unfamiliar with psychiatric care as practiced locally (Kinzie 1985). The former analysand from a coastal metropolitan area may anticipate a quite different intervention from that available in a remote resort area. Similarly, a refugee or foreign student from a developing region may expect a type of assistance different from that proffered (Tseng 1972; Odejide 1979). So long as the psychiatrist can recognize the differences in expectations, these can usually be addressed successfully—a process that has been referred to as "negotiating the illness experience" (Nichter 1981). Fortunately, these potential doctor-patient problems fall into a finite number of probable causes (Ananth 1984).

One patient expectation may consist of a focus on somatic symptoms, without attention to psychological, family, social, or cultural matters (Ludwig and Forrester 1982). This problem can generally be resolved by the following: (1) a full hearing of the somatic story, along with facilitation and clarification by the psychiatrist; (2) a medical review of symptoms of all physiological systems; and (3) a brief explanation that psychological, family, social, and cultural matters can influence health, followed by a brief initial routine inquiry into these areas.

Initial psychosocial history taking should focus on nonthreatening areas, such as community of origin, educational and occupational background, and duration of residence in the current community. Subsequent sessions can include more personal information, such as reasons for migration, disappointments since migration, and marital or intergenerational problems associated with change in residence. Migrant patients unfamiliar with the psychiatric modus operandi may be quite reluctant to provide information on an initial visit, whereas considerable personal information is usually obtainable in a second or third visit. Spending an adequate amount of time with the patient (i.e., hourly sessions) greatly aids in this process.

The patient may expect to be examined, at least in the anatomical regions where symptoms are located (Fishman 1979). Given the high prevalence of anatomical lesions among many migrant patients, this is a reasonable expectation. If the psychiatrist has seriously considered the possible biomedical dimensions of the patient's complaints, the patient is more likely to accept the psychiatrist's psychosocial interventions.

Migrant patients from rural or developing areas may interpret a passive, detached, purely interrogatory approach as evidence of physician disinterest, even hostility. Even the urban, psychologically sophisticated migrant patient—socially isolated or bereft of his or her previous social network—typically expects a more involved and supportive doctor-patient relationship. Guidance, education, suggestions, and recommendations—traditional physician attributes in most societies (Wu 1982)—are called for more often than might be the case with nonmigrants. As Kinzie (1978, 1981) has pointed out, this more active approach is even feasible when working across languages and across cultures, as with refugee patients.

Family contact should ordinarily be more intense for migrant patients, as often as every therapeutic session for outpatients or daily for hospitalized patients. Like patients themselves, migrant families are apt to be mistrustful or not to understand the psychiatric modus operandi. They may be all the more distressed at having a psychiatric disorder in the family while away from home and familiar resources—again, similar to the typical responses of patients themselves. Family systems and normative relationships vary across cultures, so rather than the common American ideal of mutually supportive independence among family members, there is an ideal of involved interdependence among family members. Family members, including even distant relatives, may serve nursing functions in treatment (e.g., administering medication, attending the patient around the clock, taking the patient on walks). Family involvement can permit certain migrant patients to be treated at home, although hospitalization might otherwise be called for (Kim 1985; Lappin and Scott 1982; Speck and Attneave 1973).

Through negotiating mutual expectations, the psychiatrist becomes an agent of acculturation for foreign migrants or resocialization for return migrants. Thus, social adjustment therapy and education occur simply through the discharges of our clinical role. Patients learn of our society and its values through us (Frank 1964). Through understanding and employing the patient's expectations, the clinician can facilitate the patient's adherence with treatment interventions and recommendations (Meichenbaum and Turk 1987).

Transference can present special problems in the care of the migrant patient. The usual transference issues (e.g., feelings toward parents, attitudes toward authority figures, relationships with people of the psychiatrist's age and sex) are modified by the patient's childhood socialization and cultural norms, so we must understand something of the patient's childhood, family, culture, and indigenous healers in order to appreciate the patient's transference issues (Hall and Bourne 1973). In addition, there may be racial, ethnic, regional, historical, and cultural dimensions to the transference (Brower 1980). That is, the patient may feel negatively or positively (or both, in various ways) depending on the physician's genetic inheritance, childhood ensocialization, and cultural affiliation—as manifested in the psychiatrist's grooming, dress, mode of relating, communication style, and evident value system. Biases of this kind may not be immediately obvious, but are often expressed indirectly.

Countertransference may also possess cultural, social, regional, or racial overtones (Bloombaum and Yamamoto 1968; Kinzie 1981; Westermeyer 1987). As with transference, the psychiatrist's attitudes and feelings are likely to have childhood, parental, and life history origins. These can present problems by being either overwhelmingly positive (e.g., revering the patient's race or culture) or negative (e.g., despising the patient's race or culture). One mode of bringing countertransference (as well as transference) matters to awareness consists of asking oneself about the history of the relationship between the patient's ethnic group and the therapist's ethnic group, along with any untoward individual events that may have occurred. War, colonialism, slavery, racism, or other conflict between the two ethnic groups can affect the doctor-patient relationship, as may personal or family traumata (e.g., assaults, rape, job loss, robbery). It can also help to recall that the therapist's culture also has concepts regarding health and illness that may conflict with those of the patient (Strassman and Galanter 1980). Countertransference issues can appear especially in work with victims of war, persecution, and terrorism (Kinzie 1985; Kinzie and Fleck 1987).

Transference and countertransference are perhaps most important when conducting psychodynamically oriented psychotherapy. Part and parcel of the therapy involves the identification and resolution (insofar as possible) of these issues. However, these issues are also important with any form of therapy requiring patient participation and compliance, including behavior modification or pharmacotherapy. If transference or countertransference seriously obstructs treatment, referral to another psychiatrist may be in order.

Selection of a language can differ during psychotherapy as compared to assessment (Marcos 1976). Earlier it was emphasized that, during assessment, one should err on the side of the patient's speaking in the primary childhood or family language in order to facilitate understanding the clinical problem. As time goes on, it may be increasingly possible for therapy to proceed in a local language that is a second language to the patient. Patient and psychiatrist may be able to develop a mutual understanding, and the clinically improving patient may be able to communicate more effectively in the local language. Therapeutic benefits to be gained from work in the local language include the following: increasing knowledge of vocabulary and grammar; acquiring ability to communicate affect in the local language; fostering acculturation, as the patient learns more of the local world view, values, and mores—

all expressed more directly and accurately in the local language than in other languages.

It can be useful to the patient and instructive for the psychiatrist to conduct therapy in both the patient's primary language and the local language, if both participants have access to both languages. Some concepts and experiences may be more readily and fully expressed in one or the other language. Events and feelings referable to the country of origin are often expressed, almost automatically, in the patient's first language. On the contrary, current events, acculturation issues, and future plans may be more readily expressed in the local language. Even the patient's choice of language may convey certain "nonverbal" or process information to the culturally sensitive psychiatrist.

During an interim phase between the patient using his or her own language and using the local language, it can be helpful to have an interpreter present for assistance as needed. If the patient cannot understand a particular question or statement made by the psychiatrist, the patient can simply glance at the interpreter for a translation. Or if the patient is unable to express a thought or feeling in the local language it can be stated to the interpreter in the patient's language. Addition of an interpreter adds to the complexity of the relationship, since both the patient's and therapist's emotional responses toward the translator, and feelings from the translator to the patient and therapist, must be considered (Acosta and Cristo 1981).

A skilled psychiatric interpreter is especially important in conducting psychotherapy (Acosta and Cristo 1981; Marcos 1976; Price 1975). Explanations for behavioral modification, instruction in self-relaxation methods, or psychodynamic interpretations all require some comprehension of psychological concepts and the ability to explain or express these clearly in the patient's language. In this context, the psychiatrist and the psychiatric translator form a team much like that of the surgeon and surgical nurse. Neither can function alone; each needs the other. A level of teamwork develops, such that each communicates rapidly, effectively, at times even nonverbally, with the other. Skilled surgeons and nurses achieve a rapid learning curve for integrated teamwork—by the fifth laparotomy, their work resembles a pair of hands operated by the same person. Similar in efficiency is the collaboration between a psychiatrist skilled in working with various interpreters in several languages, and the experienced psychiatric interpreter. Moreover, both members of the team must rely upon the skills of the other. Interpreters may not comprehend the rationale for dialogue on a particular topic, the reason for a certain question, or the plan behind a particular therapeutic interpretation; yet, they must proceed with their work based on faith in the clinician's competence. Likewise, the psychiatrist must trust the ability of the interpreter to understand the question or statement and translate it meaningfully to the patient. The interpreter must possess the confidence to question the psychiatrist regarding an unclear term or phrase, or to discuss a problematic translation with the psychiatrist.

The goals of therapy must be considered, since the patient, the family, and the psychiatrist may all have somewhat different, albeit overlapping, goals. Problems in this area can be prevented or reduced if the therapist is familiar with the patient's culture and family structure (Kinzie 1981; Tsui and Schultz 1985). For example, a refugee patient wanted respite from the ancestor ghosts that assaulted her during her sleep, and her family wanted respite from her frequent crying spells and nighttime screams. Failure of complete agreement may also occur with more sophisticated patients. For example, a recently married and relocated physician wanted treatment for her "codependence" (her father had been an alcoholic), her husband wanted a cessation to her spending sprees, and the psychiatrist wanted her to comply with medication recommendations for her affective disorder. Migrants not wishing to change their attitudes or behaviors present a special challenge, since successful treatment may require such change. Acceptance of change requires a level of surrender, giving up the past, and relinquishing previous modes of adaptation—a difficult process for all patients, but virtually impossible for some highly rigid or vulnerable patients.

Psychotherapeutic Modalities

Any type of psychotherapy employed with indigenous psychiatric patients can be employed for migrant patients. However, certain approaches and caveats are particularly relevant for migrants. These special considerations are needed in view of certain special needs, such as loss of social network, experience of highly stressful events, language obstacles, and cultural differences.

Crisis intervention and management (Jacobson et al. 1968; Lindemann 1944) can help recent migrants undergoing a recent loss or current stressor. Crisis, an inevitable aspect of migration, provides an opportunity to relinquish important aspects of the past while choosing new, more appropriate and adaptive behaviors and roles—in essence, altering oneself and one's social existence. Migrants can be assisted with crisis via the following steps:

1. Acquiring as much information as possible, including an understanding of the local implications of various losses and crises (e.g., local regulations regarding burial, means of reporting a crime, or welfare support during temporary unemployment);
2. Facilitating awareness and the expression of feeling (especially important in migrants who are so threatened by the realities of the crisis that they may ignore their own emotional response to it);
3. Suggesting alternatives for addressing the crisis (the psychiatrist may perceive alternatives not known by the migrant patient, and vice versa);
4. Employing or seeking local resources for assisting with the problem (e.g., Traveler's Aid, a private organization for helping those in need away from home; the Red Cross, which may have links to refugee camps or prisons in other coun-

tries; the Immigration and Naturalization Service of the United States Department of State; foreign embassies in Washington, D.C., and consulates in major cities);

5. Involving local and expatriate helpers or "fictive kin" (in anthropological terms), such as student advisors, refugee sponsors, and ethnic or religious agencies (e.g., Catholic Charities, Jewish Family Service, Lutheran Brotherhood);

6. Making decisions emphasizing those which are short-term, reversible, or absolutely necessary, while delaying those which are long-term or irreversible until the crisis is past;

7. Applying the PIE principles of acute management, which entail the following: Proximity = treat the person in a nearby, reasonably secure setting (i.e., do not immediately send the person back home or to a distant place); Immediacy = initiate treatment right away (i.e., do not delay until later); Expectancy = anticipate that severe symptoms are a normal reaction to tumultuous events and that most sufferers will soon be able again to cope with their lives (i.e., do not be overwhelmed by the severity of their current psychopathology).

Failure to manage a crisis appropriately can exacerbate rather than relieve problems. Keys to successful crisis management with migrants include the following:

- Complete information should be obtained prior to decision making;
- Expression of feeling should be facilitated;
- Alternatives for addressing the crisis in several ways should be reviewed and considered;
- All local community resources should be listed and considered;
- Clan elders and an available ethnic association may prove useful in addressing the situation;
- Irreversible, long-term decision making should be avoided in crisis; reversible, short-term decisions should be made until the crisis is resolving.

Kinzie et al. (1984) have warned that psychotherapy is not an entirely benign intervention in severely traumatized, terrorized, or otherwise victimized persons. Undertaken at the wrong time, or in too vigorous a fashion, or with an inappropriate patient, even gentle probing can exacerbate symptoms or precipitate more severe problems (e.g., suicide, psychosis). Facilitation and clarification should be emphasized in early stages of therapy, with probing, confrontation, and interpretation delayed until rapport is well established, the patient is improving clinically, and the psychiatrist has thorough knowledge of the case.

Some acute cases, even involving psychosis, may resolve with brief, intensive psychotherapy. These are most apt to be effective if the stressor is a major or overwhelming one and if it has occurred recently. Therapist expression of empathy, support, and close following until the patient is safely recovering can facilitate reintegration while at times obviating the need for pharmacotherapy with its attendant risks.

Crisis problems encountered among migrants often involve changing family roles, usually involving role changes regarding gender, age, and family status. This problem can manifest itself in many ways: solo mothers expecting their adolescent sons to lead the family, parents expecting their adult offspring to seek their permission for marriage or large purchases, irresponsible adolescent sons expecting their widowed mothers to hand the family finances over to them, or eldest sons (here as students or refugees) torn between remaining here and returning home when their fathers die.

Grieving death at a distance presents special problems. Funeral practices around the world serve a mental health function, by demonstrating the finality of the event (through showing, cremating, or burying the body), through evoking mutual support, via renegotiating kith and kin ties to replace obligations to and support from the deceased, and by initiating the period of grief work. The absence of a corpse and a funeral ritual undermines this culturally supported and healing process. Grief therapy may be indicated in cases of missed, complicated, or delayed grief reactions. Patients can be guided in the process of grieving by urging the following steps:

1. Undertaking an appropriate ritual despite the absence of a corpse (e.g., a Catholic mass, sitting Jewish shiva, Theravada Buddhist ceremony with prayers and "cutting strings" to the deceased);
2. Establishing a symbolic presence of the deceased for a year or longer (e.g., Asian ancestor altar, with a photograph of the deceased, his or her favorite flowers, foods, or other objects);
3. Discussing the deceased person with friends and family, reviewing the person's life, recalling happy as well as problematic events and relationships with the person.

Delayed or missed grieving of a long-past loss may present acutely. This is especially apt to occur among refugees, combat veterans, and others who have had major, ungrieved losses from months, years, or even decades ago (Baskauskas 1981). Typically these cases are precipitated by a current event.

A common theme in grief therapy with refugee veterans and Vietnam veterans is the grief and anger at loss of the country and/or the war (Munoz 1980). Survivors may perceive their sacrifices, and those of the dead colleagues, as having no meaning and having been a waste. A certain loss of innocence prevails in these patients, who—often at a young age—have trusted excessively in their military units, political leaders, or national purpose. They may have naïvely assumed that their "just cause" would necessarily win out simply on moral imperatives alone. Grief over lost innocence, misplaced trust, or naïve assumptions may also need to be addressed in grief therapy.

Another element in these missed grief cases is the relatively minor nature of the recent precipitant, at least compared to the severity of the original losses or stresses. In the case described above, the precipitant involved being laid off from work. In another example, a refugee had spent 3 years in a concentration camp, with shaming and malnutrition and a prolonged and dangerous escape from the camp (in which the escape group came under attack, and one person was killed). He developed a major depression and posttraumatic stress disorder (PTSD) when his house was burglarized and his phonograph stolen. A third refugee veteran, who had survived 20 years of war and the deaths of his wife and numerous friends in the war, developed his first major depression when years later his car was vandalized in the United States.

Behavior modification has certain advantages over one-to-one psychotherapy for immigrants and can contribute greatly to the care of these patients for several reasons. First, this modality involves relatively limited interpreter time, as compared to other forms of psychotherapy, so that non-English speakers can benefit from it. Second, it is fairly mechanistic and may be less personally threatening or laborious compared with other forms of therapy. Given a modicum of compliance, patients can improve without a culture-based faith in this modality. Third, patients and relatives can often discern some improvement within days of initiating these approaches, and so they can be motivated to persist in the treatment. Fourth, the efficacy of the treatment is usually apparent early on, so that other modalities can be initiated if the behavioral program is failing. Fifth, no direct threat to tradition, family ties, or social roles need be inherent in this method. Sixth, the principles of behavior modification are congenial to certain Buddhist, Hindu, and other practices and philosophies (De-Silva 1984; Mikulas 1978; Singh and Oberhummer 1980) and have been readily accepted by psychiatric patients in diverse cultural settings (Danquah 1982; DeRosenberg and Delgado 1985; Yamagami et al. 1982). There are also limitations to behavior modification, perhaps the main one being the limited range of symptoms and disorders for which it is effective. Nonetheless, behavior modification can—if applied thoughtfully on a specific part of the patient's problem—be used to address specific behavior problems among refugees, such as the following:

- Eating disorders, psychoactive substance use disorders, pathological gambling, other conduct disorders: treated by behavioral methods such as contingency contracting, social network/rehabilitation programs;
- Mental retardation, regressed psychiatric patients: treated by token economy;
- Panic attack, generalized anxiety, obsessive compulsive disorder, phobias, PTSD: treated by behavioral therapies such as imagery desensitization, graded stimulus desensitization, implosion or "imaginal flooding" techniques (Keane and Kaloupek 1982).

Self-relaxation techniques can aid the anxious or hypervigilant migrant patient (Buckley and Galanter 1979). As with behavior modification, it can also be beneficial across cultures and languages (Dobkin de Rios and Friedmann 1987). Audiotapes translated into the patient's language can facilitate the training process, as can Transcendental Meditation, EEG biofeedback, and other approaches. Migrants from cultures that value meditation and meditation-focused exercises (e.g., Buddhist and Hindu groups) comply especially well with this familiar modality.

Berne's "parent-adult-child" concept of human psychology (1961) can aid migrants in understanding their special dilemmas. In order to adjust to a new environment, especially one with an unfamiliar language and culture, one must learn to regress to certain childlike attitudes and behaviors, such as admitting to oneself the lack of relevant knowledge, skill, and experience in the new environment; willingness to be instructed and corrected by others (even by children), who thus become "parents" to one's own psychic "child"; taking time to play in and explore the new environment, including new activities, roles, and relationships; ability to experiment, take risks, and try new approaches and behaviors, without excessive embarrassment or injury to self-esteem; or spending considerable extra time and energy in this childlike process while also engaged in adult roles of working, homemaking, or parenting. During this adjustment period the person must avoid retreating into one's psychic "parent" as a defense. This maladaptive strategy can be manifested in the following ways: overvaluing, even unrealistically glorifying, the previous community or society; retreating into the home and family, in which the former society is rigidly overdetermined and the new environment is kept out; objecting to any evidence of the new society in one's children, spouse, relatives, or expatriate friends; becoming righteous, constantly negative, and superior acting toward the new community; or failing to make new friends among the local people or to engage in new activities.

A variety of one-to-one psychotherapies can be employed among migrants, both local and foreign born. Psychotherapeutic approaches, concepts, and techniques appropriate to migrant patients can be gleaned from Gestalt, transactional, rational-emotive, cognitive, paradoxical, psychodynamically oriented, and psychoanalytic psychotherapy. It should be borne in mind that many foreign-born, minority, and rural patients may be familiar with the notion of brief counseling (from elders, clergy, teachers, general physicians) but do not have a concept of long-term psychotherapy (with a lengthy period before notable benefit ensues). Migrant patients are thus apt to leave therapy if they do not discern some utility or benefit within a few sessions. At least for the first several sessions, some principles of short-term psychotherapy (Sifneos 1979) apply reasonably well to the initial care of these patients.

Psychotherapeutic Techniques

In working with migrants, facilitation of the patient in relating the clinical history often serves an even greater function than with local patients. Facilitation enables the psychiatrist to discern the patient's cultural values, attitudes, and norms, in addition to eliciting the clinical history and identifying psychopathological symptoms. Thorough investigation of the patient's story also enhances rapport, by demonstrating an interest in the patient and the problem. The clinician's questions can be instructive of themselves, by conveying to the patient important areas of consideration and by demonstrating the actual process of psychiatric assessment.

Clarification is also doubly important with migrant patients, since it is another means by which the clinician can learn about the patient's previous life, home, culture, and current stresses. The key to effective clarifying questions is the psychiatrist's own confusion regarding the patient's story. When confusion ensues, the patient has usually assumed that the psychiatrist shares some knowledge, experience, or attitude with the patient—when in fact, such sharing does not exist. Through clarifying the confusion, two desirable outcomes ordinarily result: the patient learns something of his or her own knowledge-experience-attitude gap with the local populace, and the psychiatrist acquires some new information about this patient in particular, and about sociocultural differences in general. This is one example of the means by which a cultural gap between patient and therapist can—like age or sex differences—enhance the therapy rather than retard it, if the therapist can be sensitive to such differences.

Empathy is an essential ingredient in much therapy with migrants. It is not conveyed through statements such as "I understand you." It may not be possible to understand completely, or even well, the feelings and experiences of many migrant patients—especially those from markedly different cultures and life-styles, or victims of unfamiliar traumas or horrors. Still, it is possible to identify with certain common human responses and to communicate this understanding to the patient via skilled therapeutic dialogue. Especially with patients who have been victimized or traumatized, the therapist must avoid the trap of confusing empathy with sympathy, approval, humoring the patient, or simple reassurances (Book 1988).

Skill at probing into the patient's thoughts, feelings, and experiences serves as an index of the therapist's ability to discern the patient's conflicts and to work effectively across cultures. Through aiding the patient to relate the story while informing the patient (through questions) of critical matters and relationships, the therapist conveys competence to and engenders trust within the patient. Even more crucial than this skill of probing is the timing of probing questions. Initiated too early in therapy, probing can delay or impede rapport. Attempted before the patient has improved sufficiently to deal with affect-laden material, probing may actually exacerbate the patient's condition and retard recovery.

Confrontation must be astutely undertaken with migrant patients. Recently arriving patients, minority patients, or those with trust problems or feelings of worthlessness may misinterpret even gentle confrontation as a rejection, and then not return to treatment. Often this intervention is needed for positive therapeutic outcome, so it should not be neglected. Methods of confronting the migrant patient without producing alienation include the following:

1. Pose the confrontation in the form of a clarification (e.g., "Can you help me understand how it is that you state 'A' but your behavior indicates 'B'?");
2. Diffuse the transference among several staff members, and assign the confrontation task to only one staff member;
3. Wait until rapport is sufficiently well established so that the patient trusts the intent of the confrontation;
4. Facilitate confrontation by family or other ethnic peers, so that the patient does not invoke racial prejudice or ethnic ignorance as a cause for the confrontation (and thereby a reason for disregarding it).

Interpretation can also pose problems in treating migrants. The psychodynamic interpretation must take into account several elements of culture. These include the patient's cultural background, the therapist's knowledge of the patient's cultural affiliations and dislikes, the nuances of the patient's cultural connotations as distinct from the therapist's cultural connotations, the patient's ability to learn and accept new insights about self and environment, and the therapist's ability to discern and to build upon the patient's awareness and maturity. The therapist must be able to weave allegory, cultural myth, world view, and hypothesized psychodynamics into interpretations that make sense to the patient yet do not threaten the patient, and at a time when the patient is ready to accept an interpretation from the indigenous stranger-therapist. As Reider (1972) has pointed out, aphorisms and metaphors can penetrate the patient's as yet unrecognized conflicts, while permitting a modicum of defensive function—allowing the patient to "titrate" the abandonment of old postures and the acquisition of new perspectives. These metaphors and allegories need not originate solely from the patient's own culture; but at least early in therapy, familiar proverbs and stories can build on old foundations. Later in therapy, use of indigenous metaphors can provide a venue to new knowledge and insight.

Interpretations should take into account, whenever possible, current events and long-past experiences. These bridging explanations in migrants fall into common categories. Predictably, one of these is cultural conflict, ensconced in the patient's own cultural preconceptions. Another involves past traumatic loss or deprivation experiences (e.g., combat, rape, torture, kidnap, terrorism) that are stirred up by some current experience. The latter may occur even several decades after the original event, which may have transpired during the patient's early life (Krell 1985).

Once rapport has been established, several techniques can be used therapeutically to promulgate a role that is more familiar to the patient. These more active techniques include the following:

1. "Homework" assignments: the patient is requested to think about a specific topic or undertake a specific action;

2. Family assignments: family members are to do something with the patient on a regular or daily basis (e.g., a 30-minute walk, a pre-bedtime massage, monitoring and administering medication);

3. Topic assignment: alerting the patient to a topic to be discussed at the next session, so that the patient (and perhaps the family) have an opportunity to consider and discuss it;

4. Therapist self-disclosure: self-disclosure by the therapist (especially if he or she has been an immigrant, lived in foreign society, been in combat, is a veteran or refugee, etc.); can be beneficial if used selectively and sparingly, keeping in mind the potential risks (e.g., that the patient feels "lectured to," or the therapist role changes to that of friend or peer rather than that of professional healer);

5. Physical examination (e.g., of a painful limb or scar) or touching a hand or forearm (e.g, during an abreaction) can enhance transference but can also be threatening depending on the patient's diagnosis (e.g., paranoia), culture, and sex; until the therapist is more knowledgeable about the patient, it is best to have others in the room, to ask the patient's permission (e.g., to examine an old wound or torture scar), and to avoid male-female touching until one is aware of the patient's cultural norms in this regard (e.g., some Islamic and Hindu sects proscribe any cross-sex touching by a non-spouse or by non-kin, even by a physician; male Buddhist monks in some sects may not touch or be touched by a woman).

Psychiatrists not trained in psychoanalysis encounter migrant patients who have been former psychoanalytic patients elsewhere. These patients can be rewarding or problematic to treat, depending on the circumstance. If the patient expects a psychiatrist to resume psychoanalytic treatment, or the non-analyst attempts to do so, the results are virtually assured to turn out badly. However, many of these patients can do well with other forms of therapy besides psychoanalysis. Typically, these patients have made adequate adjustments and have recurrent problems only when some stress is encountered, such as the migration itself, or a marriage or a failure while away from home. These patients often respond well to crisis intervention and brief or time-limited psychotherapy. If it appears that a resumption of psychoanalysis is warranted, they should be referred to a trained analyst. As with all patients, any therapeutic recommendations must be based on careful assessment. A history of receiving psychoanalysis is no guarantee against subsequent development of another psychiatric disorder for which psychoanalysis may or may not be clinically appropriate.

Some migrants are prone not to relate emotional material or experiences. This is especially apt to occur among PTSD patients, various victims (i.e., of torture, sexual assault, combat, terrorism), somatizing patients, suspicious or mistrustful patients, illiterate patients, and those with limited education or limited cross-cultural experience before migration. These same patients, if having moderately severe depression or anxiety, frequently have troubling dreams or nightmares. These sleep experiences can provide considerable grist for the therapeutic mill, as well as aid the clinician in assessing and in evaluating the results of therapy. Migrant patients who are strongly blocked on recognizing and/or expressing their own feelings or concerns are generally willing to describe their dreams in great detail with much associated affect. The following relevant dream information should be obtained:

- Content of the patient's dreams or nightmares;
- Recurrent themes that pervade several different dreams (e.g., ancestor dreams, previous combat experiences, escapist dreams, being chased or threatened);
- Identity of characters in the dream (e.g., specific living or dead persons, enemy soldiers, ghosts of a particular age or sex);
- Location and timing of the dream (i.e., refugees and combat veterans with PTSD are apt to dream of events from years ago on another continent; those with here-and-now crisis

problems are apt to dream about recent events occurring close to home);
- Frequency of the dream (i.e., several times per night has a different significance from monthly or anniversary dreams, which many refugees and combat veterans can tolerate without disability or care-seeking);
- Intensity and consequences of the dream (e.g., some patients may merely wake up and go back to sleep immediately, while others are agitated for hours and are fearful of falling back to sleep);
- Meaning ascribed by the patient to the dream (e.g., this varies from those who view dreams as preternatural but actual events occurring in the "dream" or "sleep" world, to those who view dreams merely as the neurotransmitter effluvia of one's REM sleep cycles serving to clear the frontal lobes of unneeded data stored temporarily);
- Affect attached to the dream (e.g., one refugee veteran— unemployed and receiving welfare—savored his combat dreams, which served to vent his rage at his conquering enemy and to reaffirm his former identity as a strong and courageous leader of men; another refugee veteran, on losing his job, was assaulted in his dreams by combat scenes in which the ghosts of his dead comrades would rise out of their bodies to chase and terrify him).

Affective reexperiencing of traumatic, stressful, humiliating, or loss events can be a key therapeutic step in treating some cases of PTSD, depression, and phobic and obsessive compulsive disorders — especially when these are associated with somatization. The first step lies in deciding whether the patient is ready to undertake this stressful treatment. For example, a psychotic Cambodian refugee was prematurely treated with affective reexperiencing alone at a "torture victim rehabilitation center" with disastrous results, precipitating a suicide attempt and exacerbation of her psychosis. If the patient is deemed ready, the therapist facilitates the patient in a full expression of the traumatic events. Adequate time should be set aside for this process, especially for the first interview (about 1–2 hours). If the patient does not live with concerned others, hospitalization may be required to ensure support. Facilitation should be the primary technique during the initial session, with only limited clarification. Confrontation or interpretation must be delayed until later sessions. Patients' affective states can vary from a controlled, white-knuckle recitation of the facts, to a highly emotional abreaction. Generally, the telling is accompanied by animation, agitation, excitement, and considerable affect (e.g., anger, remorse, sadness). Therapists who are inexperienced or unaccustomed to this work may have difficulty in dealing with this initial phase. Pitfalls include redirecting the patient toward a less stressful subject, becoming emotionally distraught, merely sympathizing with or reassuring the patient, or employing inappropriate techniques (e.g., excessive clarification, premature interpretation), or pushing the patient to tell more (Parson 1985), rather than facilitating a full expression of the event or events at the patient's own pace. This "telling" phase can in itself be therapeutic, especially if the patient has been attempting to push it out of awareness, has kept it as a private secret, has been rebuffed by friends or relatives when trying to relate it, or if the patient carries considerable shame, guilt, or humiliation regarding the event.

Once the horrific events have been related in one or a few sessions, it is possible to proceed with the next step, affective relearning. This takes place via a detailed re-exploration of the events. At this phase, the primary therapeutic technique is clarification, in which the therapist asks detailed questions about the patient's thoughts and feelings concerning the events at the time (insofar as these can be resurrected retrospectively) and at the current time. This process permits the identification of unrealistic expectations of self, over-responsibility, missed grief, and personally unacceptable thoughts or feelings (e.g., longing for certain aspects of combat, prison, or concentration camp life). During this phase, patients often become more acutely aware of their feelings in the here and now, so that events of the past can be related to current events. For example, a Vietnamese torture victim was reunited with his family after a decade. Over a period of several months he developed a melancholic depression. After first being assisted in relating the horrors to which he was subjected, he was then able to recognize that he actually missed certain aspects of being in prison—in particular, the mutual support and understanding and the close comradeship that he shared with fellow inmates. Since reuniting with his family, he had not been able to reestablish a similar close feeling with his family in the United States. During the clarification phase, as his sensitivity to his own feelings emerged, he was able to recognize his own concerns about the personal and cultural changes in his children and wife in the United States—some of which he admired and some of which he eschewed.

At the next step in this type of therapy, cognitive restructuring may be beneficial (Beck et al. 1979). Interpretation, confrontation, and education are primary techniques in this process. Certain common themes are encountered at this phase, such as the following:

- Omnipotence manifested by feelings of overresponsibility in parents, clan leaders, and military or militia leaders: this results in the patient's feeling responsible for violence or losses over which the patient had no control, with subsequent shame and self-blame;
- Omniscience manifested by the self-expectation that governmental overthrow, military attack, or violence during refugee flight should have been foreseen and avoided: this results in guilt for ensuing losses and violent consequences;
- Escapism to the past, while ignoring challenges in the difficult present: these patients obsess on reveries of past times in which the patient or group manifested their competence (e.g., wishing to return to the war, refugee flight, guerrilla activities) (Solursh 1988);
- Persistence of naïve wishes or fantasies about the world as a predictable, safe, and controllable environment in which

all sacrifices or pain are meaningful: these patients alternately fear that there is no justice, security, or predictability
anywhere in the world, so that any event that intrudes on
this fantasy-fear duality (e.g., theft, vandalism, losing a job)
can have reactive consequences well in excess of their apparent stress.

These matters are of course not unique to migrants, although they are frequent among such groups as combat veterans, refugees, and hostages. For example, rape victims and
the families and friends of local homicide victims must also
deal not only with the loss of the relative, but also with mul-
tiple other losses, such as the loss of the illusion of invulner-
ability, loss of trust in the community and the police, and
the lost view of a totally just world in which perpetrators are
necessarily punished (Masters et al. 1988; Roth and Lebowitz
1988). Among victims of persecution and disaster survivors,
these cognitive maladies exist among hundreds, and even thousands of people. Besides cognitive restructuring, sociotherapies
and certain public health strategies (covered in Chapter 8) can
be beneficial.

Education assumes a central part in the therapy of many
migrant patients. Unfamiliar with local customs, laws, and
procedures, they can get into social dilemmas more readily
and then experience more difficulty in extricating themselves
from these problems. As with other therapeutic interventions,
education to the realities of the current environment (sometimes harsh or difficult to accept) should be delayed for an
appropriate phase of treatment.

Role play is an effective means for identifying problematic
attitudes and for teaching new skills. Role play may focus
on numerous new and unfamiliar social transactions: e.g., applying for a job, confronting a co-worker regarding racist
remarks, discussing an interfamily problem concerning a neighbor, or reporting a crime to the police. Rehearsing the interaction can aid the patient in overcoming excessive fear or sup-
pressing disruptive anger, in order to deal effectively with the

problem at hand. Videotapes of the role-play situation can reduce the interfering emotional response and provide positive feedback for learning new skills. If role play is used in a group setting with several migrant patients, considerable vicarious learning may ensue from addressing problems encountered by many migrants.

Special Issues

Coping mechanisms adaptive in the old residence may be problematic or nonadaptive in the new setting. For example, total reliance on the clan or ethnic group may have been appropriate in the past, but inadequate in the United States. Close association with family in times of severe illness or death could be feasible when the family lived close by, but it is not consistent with continued use if the family lives hundreds of miles away. In order to cope with the new problems posed by migration, the migrant must alter some coping mechanisms, abandon others, and learn still new ones. Entirely new coping mechanisms may be needed to cope with unfamiliar experiences, such as racism, changing personality and family identity, ethnic prejudice, new social mores, an unfamiliar legal and political system, or communication problems.

Risk taking is an inherent aspect of adaptation to a new environment and learning new coping styles (e.g., obtaining a job, acquiring new friends, undertaking new recreational activities). This creates an inherent conflict, since we are generally reluctant to assume a risk (which per se entails a possibility of failure) unless we are reasonably secure and able to accept a failure without excessive threat to self-esteem, or we are so pushed *ad extremis* that a risk must be taken, even if the outcome poses a serious threat to self-esteem or to survival. Migrants must undertake numerous small and large risks over a prolonged period. The greater the cultural gap, the less experienced the individual in cross-cultural living, the less secure and the more limited the resources, then the greater is the risk of failing. Migrants need to experience both successes and failures as a result of their risk taking. Successes reinforce self-esteem and provide migrants with the feedback that they are taking reasonable risks and pursuing achievable goals. Occasional failures are needed also to inform migrants of their limitations and areas requiring more knowledge, effort, or experience. Until migrant patients are reasonably secure and recovered, they should be guided toward risk taking in which the chance of failure is small, and the consequences of failure are temporary and not devastating. Later, with security and good self-esteem, risk taking can involve larger risks of failure and more lasting consequences.

Migrants have been said to become 150% people in order to adjust and survive well. That is, the 100% adaptive effort sufficient for existence in one's home environment is insufficient for the migrant. Depending on the cultural gap, the migrant must rebuild a new social network, learn new customs and skills, and perhaps acquire a new language. In terms of cultural distance, one might be able to think of needing to be a 120% person if one is moving from a rural area to a nearby city, or a 200% person if one is moving to a totally different country with unfamiliar language, religion, and political system. Even with this effort the migrant may end up marginal to one or both societies (Park 1928), unless the two societies are reasonably congenial to each other or the migrant is able to transcend the differences intact.

An additional dimension not reflected in the "150% person" is the inherent conflict that occurs between the mores and regulations of the home society and the resettlement society. People may have to maintain one set of values at home and another set of values at school or work. The timing of this conflict can vary, depending on the nature of the two cultures. For example, most American Indian and black American children perform well in elementary school, apparently being able to balance effectively the expectations of home and school. As peer influences grow in importance during preteen and early teen years, academic performance plummets and the school drop-out rate soars. Many children in these two minority groups fail to meet the conflicting values and expectations set by their peers and families vis-à-vis those set by school authorities. Of interest, in other health areas not influenced by peers, such as dental care, these groups show good compliance with healthy prevention practices (Cipes et al. 1983). Conversely, preteen and adolescent Asian American children have little trouble in coping with the expectation of peers, family, and school during this time. Later in college or university, however, Asian American students may not be able to achieve the high goals set by parents or family, given the standards or competition at that level.

Out of these inherent conflicts, several alternative pathways exist. One alternative is to opt out of the field and flee in some apparently less-stressful direction (e.g., underachievement, drop out, unemployment, welfare dependence). Another alternative lies in sublimating in one or both cultures—i.e., becoming an outstanding "hyphenated-American," or expatriate community leader, or perhaps even both. A third path lies in consciously recognizing, negotiating, and compromising the demands of the two cultures or communities. A fourth option consists of changing both the donor culture and the recipient society in ways congenial to the migrants (long part of the American tradition). The resolution of this inherent conflict leads to diverse positive and negative outcomes: a high casualty rate among migrants, the evaluation of new lifestyles, a virtual explosion of diverse personality styles, and innovative cultural developments. Psychiatrists treating migrant patients can participate in the creative process, while being challenged to engage creatively in the psychotherapeutic process (Rothenberg 1988).

On an individual as well as a community basis, this conflict can lead to acculturation or ghettoization. Those able to become a 150% person, with the strength to sublimate and compromise and with the ability to recognize and create, can achieve some functional level of acculturation in the majority society. Those unable to reach this goal fall back to a "ghetto" position— "ghetto" not necessarily in the geographic-historical sense of ghetto, but in the psychological sense of an embattled, defensive, inner-directed, and internally supported life-style that ignores the reality of the surrounding and dominant society. Commonly the transition from ghettoization to acculturation proceeds over several generations. Thus, some second-generation citizens have few acculturation tasks to perform since their parents have done much of the adjustment. Yet, other third-generation citizens can face a tremendous acculturation task if their parents and grandparents survived by assuming a "ghetto" outlook.

Self-esteem and identity issues exist for many migrants, native and foreign, voluntary and involuntary. People derive at least a part of their identity from their region, town, neighborhood, and social network. Migration removes these connections to some greater or lesser extent, leaving the individual with a kind of psychic wound. Closely allied with identity, self-esteem may likewise be dealt a temporary blow. One is not so competent, familiar, and efficient in the new place. Even simple needs may require extraordinary measures for a time. To learn the new system, perhaps even a new language, the migrant must regress to a childlike dependence on others, a willingness to be instructed and corrected, and an acceptance of younger and less knowledgeable instructors (Carlin 1986; Naditch and Morrissey 1976).

The integration of diverse therapies in the same patient, including more than one psychotherapy and other therapies (i.e., somatotherapies, sociotherapies), is part of most psychiatrists' daily tasks. Ordinarily this integration presents no greater inherent problem for migrants than for other patients. Those treating numerous migrants must be prepared to apply a diversity of therapies in the same patient and to phase them appropriately, while not overtaxing the patient's and family's ability to participate in the treatment process. As Karasu (1987) has observed, medication often takes effect sooner and has more rapid observable effects than psychotherapy, which often has more delayed results. However, the benefits of psychotherapy are often more apt to persist, especially in the interpersonal and social dimensions—the latter being especially critical areas for many migrant patients.

It can be valuable for those conducting cross-cultural psychotherapy to be aware of therapies employed in other cultures (Ikema 1979). These are sometimes referred to as *culture bound,* but they are more properly termed *culture-related* psychotherapy since the methods are not so much unique as over determined in the parent culture. For example, *morita* therapy in Japan (prescribed in the early care of certain severe nonpsychotic conditions) involves considerable instruction, direction, and suggestion by the psychiatrist in a context of social isolation, regression, and intense nursing care by one nurse (Chang 1974; Ishiyama 1986). Some Thai psychiatrists prescribe Buddhist meditative exercises or a period of temporary monkhood in a Buddhist monastery at certain phases of specific disorders. *Cuento* or folktale therapy, developed for Puerto Rican children, consists of employing local folktales to identify local and American values with which the patients must cope (Constantino et al. 1986). Knowledge of these modalities can aid the psychiatrist in planning treatment and in guiding patients in their own culturally consistent recovery activities (e.g., healing rituals, "warrior re-entry" ceremonies for American Indian combat veterans, Catholic confession). For literate patients, bibliotherapy—writing an autobiography of past events, or keeping a diary of current events, can contribute to greater emotional control and cognitive self-awareness.

References

Acosta FX, Cristo MH: Development of bilingual interpreter program: an alternative model for Spanish-speaking services. Professional Psychology 12:474–481, 1981

Ananth J: Treatment of immigrant Indian patients. Can J Psychiatry 29:490–493, 1984

Baskauskas L: The Lithuanian refugee experience and grief. International Migration Review 15:276–291, 1981

Beck AT, Rush AJ, Shaw BF, et al: Cognitive Therapy of Depression. New York, Guilford, 1979

Berne E: Transactional Analysis in Psychotherapy. New York, Grove Press, 1961

Bloombaum M, Yamamoto J: Cultural stereotyping among psychotherapists. J Consult Clin Psychol 32:99, 1968

Book HE: Empathy: misconceptions and misuses in psychotherapy. Am J Psychiatry 145:420–424, 1988

Brower IC: Counseling Vietnamese. Personnel Guidance Journal 58:646–652, 1980

Buckley P, Galanter M: Altered states of consciousness during psychotherapy: a historical and cultural perspective. Int J Soc Psychiatry 25:118–124, 1979

Carlin J: Child and adolescent refugees: psychiatric assessment and treatment, in Refugee Mental Health in Resettlement Countries. Edited by Williams CL, Westermeyer J. Washington, DC, Hemisphere, 1986, pp 131–139

Chang SC: Morita therapy. Am J Psychother 28:208–221, 1974

Cipes MH, Kegeles SS, Lund AK, et al: Differences in dental experiences, practices, and beliefs of inner-city and suburban adolescents. Am J Public Health 73:1305–1309, 1983

Constantino G, Malgady RG, Rogler LH: Cuento therapy: a culturally sensitive modality for Puerto Rican children. J Consult Clin Psychol 54:639–645, 1986

Danquah SA: The practice of behavior therapy in West Africa: the case in Ghana. J Behav Ther Exp Psychiatry 13:5–13, 1982

DeRosenberg FK, Delgado F: The establishment of a behavior therapy unit within a general hospital in Venezuela: the first five years. J Behav Ther Exp Psychiatry 16:5–7, 1985

DeSilva P: Buddhism and behavior modification. Behav Res Ther 6:661–678, 1984

Dobkin de Rios M, Friedmann JK: Hypnotherapy with Hispanic burn patients. Int J Clin Exp Hypn 35:87–94, 1987

Fishman RG: Spiritualism in Western New York: a study in ritual healing. Med Anthropol 3:1–22, 1979

Frank JD: Persuasion and Healing: A Comparative Study of Psychotherapy. Baltimore, MD, Johns Hopkins University Press, 1964

Hall AL, Bourne PG: Indigenous therapists in a Southern Black urban community. Arch Gen Psychiatry 28:137–142, 1973

Ikema Y: Eastern and Western approaches to self-regulation. Can J Psychiatry 24:471–480, 1979

Ishiyama FI: Morita therapy: its basic features and cognitive intervention for anxiety treatment. Psychotherapy 23:375–381, 1986

Karasu TB: The psychotherapy of the future. Psychosomatics 28:380–384, 1987

Keane TM, Kaloupek DG: Imaginal flooding in the treatment of a posttraumatic stress disorder. J Consult Clin Psychol 50:138–140, 1982

Kim SC: Family therapy for Asian Americans: a strategic-structural framework. Psychotherapy 22:342–348, 1985

Kinzie JD: Lessons from cross-cultural psychotherapy. Am J Psychother 32:510–520, 1978

Kinzie JD: Evaluation and psychotherapy of Indochinese refugee patients. Am J Psychother 35:251–261, 1981

Kinzie JD: Cultural aspects of psychiatric treatment with Indochinese refugees. American Journal of Social Psychiatry 5:47–53, 1985

Kinzie JD, Fleck J: Psychotherapy with severely traumatized refugees. Am J Psychother 41:82–94, 1987

Kinzie JD, Frederikson RH, Toth B, et al: Posttraumatic stress disorder among survivors of Cambodian concentration camps. Am J Psychiatry 141:645–650, 1984

Krell R: Child survivors of the Holocaust: 40 years later. J Am Acad Child Psychiatry 24:378–380, 1985

Jacobson GF, Strickler M, Morley WE: Generic and individual approaches to crisis intervention. Am J Public Health 58:338–343, 1968

Lappin J, Scott S: Intervention in a Vietnamese refugee family, in Ethnicity and Family Therapy. Edited by McGoldrich M, Pearce JK, Giordano J. New York, Guilford, 1982

Lindemann E: Symptomatology and management of acute grief. Am J Psychiatry 101:141–148, 1944

Ludwig AM, Forrester RL: Nerves, but not mentally. J Clin Psychiatry 43:187–190, 1982

Marcos LR: Bilinguals in psychotherapy: language as an emotional barrier. Am J Psychother 30:552–560, 1976

Masters R, Friedman LN, Getzel G: Helping families of homicide victims: a multidimensional approach. Journal of Traumatic Stress 1:109–125, 1988

Meichenbaum D, Turk DC: Facilitating Treatment Adherence. New York, Plenum, 1987

Mikulas WL: Four noble truths of Buddhism related to behavior therapy. Psychological Record 28:59–67, 1978

Munoz L: Exile as bereavement: socio-psychological manifestations of Chilean exiles in Great Britain. Br J Med Psychol 53:227–232, 1980

Naditch MP, Morrissey RF: Role stress, personality, and psychopathology in a group of immigrant adolescents. J Abnorm Psychol 83:113–118, 1976

Nichter M: Negotiation of the illness experience: Ayurvedic therapy and the psychosocial dimension of illness. Cult Med Psychiatry 5:5–24, 1981

Odejide AO: Traditional (native) psychiatric practice: its role in modern psychiatry in a developing country. Psychiatric Journal of the University of Ottawa 4:297–301, 1979

Park RE: Human migration and the marginal man. American Journal of Sociology 6:881–893, 1928

Parson ER: Ethnicity and traumatic stress: the intersecting point in psychotherapy, in Trauma and Its Wake. Edited by Figley CR. New York, Brunner-Mazel, 1985, pp 314–337

Pedersen P: The intercultural context of counseling and therapy, in Cultural Conceptions of Mental Health and Therapy. Edited by Marsella AJ, White GM. Boston, MA, Reidel, 1982, pp 333–358

Price J: Foreign language interpreting in psychiatric practice. Aust N Z J Psychiatry 9:263–267, 1975

Reider N: Metaphor as interpretation. Int J Psychoanal 53:463–469, 1972

Roth S, Lebowitz L: The experience of sexual trauma. Journal of Traumatic Stress 1:79–107, 1988

Rothenberg A: The Creative Process of Psychotherapy. New York, Norton, 1988

Sifneos PE: Short-Term Dynamic Psychotherapy. New York, Plenum, 1979

Singh R, Oberhummer I: Behavior therapy within a setting of Karma Yoga. J Behav Ther Exp Psychiatry 11:135–141, 1980

Solursh L: Combat addiction: post-traumatic stress disorder re-explored. Psychiatric Journal of the University of Ottawa 13:17–20, 1988

Speck RV, Attneave CL: Family Networks. New York, Pantheon, 1973

Strassman RJ, Galanter M: The Abhidharma: a cross-cultural model for the psychiatric application of medication. Int J Soc Psychiatry 26:293–299, 1980

Tseng WS: Psychiatric study of shamanism in Taiwan. Arch Gen Psychiatry 26:561–565, 1972

Tseng WS, McDermott JF: Psychotherapy: historical roots, universal elements, and cultural variations. Am J Psychiatry 132:378–384, 1975

Tsui P, Schultz GL: Failure of rapport: why psychotherapeutic engagement fails in the treatment of Asian clients. Am J Orthopsychiatry 55:561–569, 1985

Westermeyer J: Clinical considerations in cross cultural diagnosis. Hosp Community Psychiatry 38:160–165, 1987

Wu DYH: Psychotherapy and emotion in traditional Chinese medicine, in Cultural Conceptions of Mental Health and Therapy. Edited by Marsella AJ, White GM. Boston, MA, Reidel, 1982, pp 285–301

Yamagami T, Okuma H, Morinaga Y, et al: Practice of behavior therapy in Japan. J Behav Ther Exp Psychiatry 13:21–26, 1982

Chapter 8
Sociotherapies

Chapter 8

Sociotherapies

Family Therapy

Family therapy often presents unusual challenges in the care of migrant patients. Not all members of the family may have migrated; the person may even be without any local relatives. Absent family members can still exert strong influence on the patient through phone calls, letters, financial support, or traditional loyalties. The patient's cultural definition of who comprises a family may differ from that of the psychiatrist. For example, in a strongly patriarchal/patrilocal culture, the wife's relatives may not be considered "family" while the husband's father, uncles, and brothers may be considered close family members—and vice versa in strongly matriarchal/matrilocal societies. Across cultures, families also differ in willingness to discuss family matters with a stranger, including a physician. This can be circumvented by caucus family therapy: i.e., discussing the matter with several family members individually or in subgroups (Kim 1985), although this adds to the time and laboriousness of dealing with family issues. This Byzantine approach does contribute to the development of rapport and may not be necessary once the clinician has rapport with the family (Lappin and Scott 1982), but junior family members may still not be willing or able to speak freely in the presence of a culturally supported matriarch or patriarch. With strongly matriarchal or patriarchal families, an eventual family meeting may resemble more a formal family affirmation of decisions already reached in a series of smaller "caucus" meetings, in which the compromises have already been negotiated. Psychologist Attneave (herself part American Indian) and her co-workers have employed extended family methods or family-network therapy (which can last 3 or 4 hours per session) with good effect (Speck and Attneave 1973). The absent-family therapy approach consists of addressing family problems in individual or group therapy (i.e., in the absence of other family members) with the aim of enhancing family strength and mutual support, and effecting positive family change. All of these methods, and other creative alternatives as well, should be considered in dealing with the migrant family. Families themselves may have notions regarding how best to proceed.

Certain of Berne's gamesmanship notions (1961) apply well for problematic family responses to psychopathology. Migrant families are especially apt to engage in "rescuing," "enabling," and "persecutory" behaviors with a psychiatrically ill member. Several factors associated with migration contribute to this common phenomenon. The family may not be aware of other resources available in the community, and so erroneously conclude that the family alone must remedy the situation. Some families are aware of the local resources but do not trust them to assist with the problem. More than the nonmigrant families, the migrant family may minimize the severity of the clinical problem. Family members, who have encountered their own migration-related distress, may misperceive even severe psychopathology as being qualitatively similar to their own adjustment—when in fact there may be very little resemblance between their own anxiety or depressive symptoms and the patient's mania or schizophrenia. Families may blame themselves for the patient's condition, believing that the migration may have produced the disorder (which may be partially true from an epidemiological perspective, but which can seldom be proven in any one case). Families coming from areas with poor or nonexistent social, health, and mental health services may perceive no other alternative than their own repeatedly ineffectual interventions. Examples of behaviors often encountered among migrants include the following:

• Enabling: continuing to provide an alcohol- or drug-abusing family member with resources to purchase alcohol or drugs (Szapocznik et al. 1978a);

- Rescuing: intervening when a manic, schizophrenic, or character-disordered relative repeatedly gets into trouble with authorities;
- Persecuting: severely punishing the difficult child who has attention deficit disorder, a learning disability, or an organic brain syndrome.

The current welfare system often functions to "enable" certain migrant families (especially refugees and mentally ill migrants) in maladaptive behavior, especially isolative withdrawal from the new society and abuse of alcohol or drugs. Repeated "rescuing" by sponsors and relocation counselors can undermine the motivation to cope with changes, although change itself is a "traditional" feature of this society. Monitoring by the welfare agents can become a "persecutory" pastime, in which the worker actively pushes the individual who passively resists these efforts.

The issues of translation, interpretation, meaning, and symbolism exist for the cross-cultural treatment of families, as they do for individuals. Tseng (1985) has pointed up some of the differences in families and family styles that should be considered in assessment and treatment (e.g., cultural definitions of family, distribution of power and authority in the family, cultural rules of family obligation and exchange). Books have been published on family therapy as conducted in various cultures (Kaslow 1982) and on family treatment approaches with particular ethnic groups (McGoldrich et al. 1982). These latter resources can be helpful in sensitizing the clinician to family culture matters, but cannot be applied whole-cloth or stereotypically to all migrant family cases. As with individuals, migrant families undergo changes with migration. These family changes can involve structure (often going from "more extended" to "more nuclear" family organization), function, modes of relating and communicating, loyalties, and expectations.

PSYCHIATRIC CARE OF MIGRANTS

Group Therapy

Group therapy can be employed among migrants, albeit with some modifications and limitations. Some ethnic groups are not accustomed to self-disclosure, especially of personal weaknesses, in a group setting. The self-disclosure necessary in group therapy may be viewed by these migrants as overly self-centered, attention seeking, or pessimistic. For example, a group of recovering American Indian alcoholics avoided "confession" of their misdeeds while drinking, although they readily reported their "close calls" in dangerous situations, the harm that befell others in the drinking group, and alternatives that they had found to recreational drinking. Migrants who share common readjustment tasks often function well in group sessions, such as refugee solo mothers, torture or disaster victims, combat veterans, unaccompanied refugee adolescents, or those adolescent refugees in solo parent homes. This modality generally requires that the leader or leaders as well as the patient speak a common language; it can be done with an interpreter (such as for instructional purposes), but this greatly delays the group interactions. Participants may tolerate a group interpreter for a session or two, but not permanently. One alternative is to assign the interpreter to the one member of the group who does not speak the language (typically leader or supervisor), thereby allowing the group to proceed at its own pace. Group therapy leaders must understand much more about the patients' culture and life experience than individual therapists, since the latter can more readily interrupt the one-to-one discussion in order to clarify a particular point, without necessarily disrupting the flow of the therapy.

Bibliotherapy as well as art, music, dance-movement, and recreational therapies, when conducted in groups, have special utility with certain migrants. Art work can aid children; torture, combat, or hostage victims; those unable to express their feelings in the local language; and those who fear loss of control in expressing their feelings (Brower 1980). Migrant adolescents may vent their feelings more comfortably, confidently, and poignantly in music and lyrics, than in therapy. Even illiterate migrants can render their feelings in the stance and movement of exercise-dance therapy, without the need to know the local language. Certain community activities, such as preparing for and giving a ceremonial dinner, can be undertaken with much language-free cooperation. Certain recreational activities and sports have the same advantage (e.g., gardening, attending a sports event or concert, hiking, sailing). Writing down one's dreams or one's day-to-day experiences can also contribute to other therapies.

"Mutual help" groups have had good effect on patients who have experienced major losses (Marmar et al. 1988). This approach has been most usefully applied to families undergoing specific kinds of losses, such as the homicide of a family member (Masters et al. 1988) and adjustments such as acculturation (Szapocznik and Kurtines 1980; Szapocznik et al. 1980, 1984). For example, the following groups share common migrational adjustment dilemmas: out-of-state medical students just entering medical school; solo-mother refugees, whose husbands were killed in war or were in prison camps, and who tend to underacculturate; eldest adolescent sons who are refugees in the United States, whose fathers have died or are in concentration camps, and who tend to be at odds with their mothers; American Indian alcoholics from rural reservation areas, attempting to adopt a sober life in an urban setting; cross-racial adoptive parents and their Korean-born adopted children; and minors placed in foster homes because their parents are mentally ill.

Marmar et al. (1988) have shown a greater attrition from the "mutual help" group modality compared to one-to-one treatment. However those who persisted in the "mutual help" group showed significant improvement in symptom self-report [on the 90-item Symptom Checklist (SCL-90) and Beck Depression Inventory]. A combination of one-to-one and group therapies for migrants appears to be most successful, especially if some patients further along in their adjustment can act as role models or guides for newer patients.

Social-Network Reconstruction

Not all migrant patients require help with social-network reconstruction. Certain migrant patients do need such help, however. These include those who have recently arrived, have previously been unable to acquire an adequate social network, or possess a pathogenic social network (e.g., alcoholics, drug abusers, gamblers, thieves, delinquents). Those who require special assistance in this area first need education in the mental health benefits of a sufficiently large, diverse, long-lasting, and reciprocal social network. Next, they must be aware of the obstacles to establishing a new social network. Finally, it is necessary to coach most migrant patients as they build a network.

One obstacle to social-network reconstruction lies in the fact that, at any one point in time, most people have an adequately sized social network. In order to meet the reciprocal demands of the network, one cannot add new members indefinitely. This factor that naturally inhibits larger and larger networks works against the migrant seeking to recreate a network. It means that the migrant, in attempting to establish friendships, must take repeated chances of being rebuffed.

A potential trap for migrants lies in entering relationships with local people who themselves need relationships because of their own problems with interpersonal relationships. Migrants thus may establish relationships with character-disordered, substance-abusing, or otherwise disabled people. Migrants are also at risk to being taken advantage of by persons who prey on lonely or naïve migrants.

Migrants can be guided toward persons or organizations in which the risks of rejection, entrapment, or manipulation are reduced. A partial list of options for migrants includes: approaching new neighbors and co-workers, who typically have "lost" the neighbor or co-worker whom the migrant has replaced and thus may have a "spare niche" in their own social networks; joining an expatriate association or church group, in which the task of the leaders is to welcome new persons

Sociotherapies

and to facilitate their entry into the group; joining local associations, sports or hobby groups, or organizations in which the migrant shares interests, skills, or identity with other members; and seeking out other congenial migrants who share the same need for social-network reconstruction. Counsel should focus on fostering groups with a shared interest in mutual activity (in social-network jargon, "plexus groups"). These groups vary with age, sex, and station in life. Each subgroup usually contains a few to several persons, unified around a common identity or activity as in the following examples: face-to-face living group (e.g., family of origin, family of marriage, roommates); relatives who are seen regularly (e.g., holidays, family rituals), sometimes replaced by "fictive kin" (nonrelatives who assume the roles of relatives); special friends who share a major occupational identity, such as among co-workers, fellow students, the local "coffee klatch" of homemakers; friends who share a common activity or avocation (e.g., playing cards, hunting, a handicraft); and associates in a formal group or organization (e.g., political party, professional guild, expatriate organization).

Pitfalls or danger signs exist in social-network reconstruction. One-to-one plexus groups (i.e., the patient and one other person) tend to be unstable, especially when the other person does not know anyone else in the network. Too small a network (e.g., only one or two plexus groups) makes the individual overly dependent on an excessively small group, so that any temporary problem or disruption can be overly distressful. Lack of reciprocity—either total giving or total receiving—is evidence of immature social relationships (i.e., a need for an exclusive "parent" or "child" role). An ever-changing network augurs against the development of loyalty, reciprocity, and persistence through difficult times.

Patience is needed in the development of a new network. A solid, reliable, and supportive network cannot be re-created within months; a few to several years are needed. A certain minimal level of congeniality among most network members is desirable, since—even though in different plexus groups—

213

they still encounter one another through their shared "possession" or "investment" in the proband. It is through one another's social networks that we reach a much larger number of acquaintances than we can personally sustain in our own "intimate social network." Most adults have close reciprocal relationships with only 20–30 people, but can name about 1,500 people whom they know personally.

The social network, and its associated obligations, is largely lost through migrations. This permits the individual to have enough time and energy to reconstruct the network, as well as time and energy for new tasks (e.g., college, a new job). Loneliness, the need for friends and associates, and striving after social roles and identities provides motivation. Available time and need drives this sometimes difficult effort. Our clinical role as psychiatrists lies in understanding and guiding this natural or "healing" process.

Social Strategies in the Desensitization of Phobias

Migration can and should give rise to certain concerns and insecurities. Until one can recognize and avoid local dangers, one's person and property are at risk. Uncommonly insecure, anxious, mistrustful, or socially unskilled persons can become disabled by excessive worries and fears. These anxieties tend to feed on themselves in a downward spiral, as more fear leads to more isolation, and greater isolation leads to more fear. Reversal of this process can require a major therapeutic effort in the migrant patient.

Phobias in migrant patients are predominantly social phobias and agoraphobia, although acrophobia, claustrophobia, and other forms can arise. Among combat veterans and refugees, phobic symptoms may appear with night, fireworks, funerals, or violent movies and television programs. Unfamiliar experiences or contexts, such as traffic jams, high buildings or bridges, elevators, or escalators (in rural or third-world migrants) can likewise give rise to specific phobias. In many migrants, these

214

symptoms are transient, not disabling, and tend to resolve over weeks or months.

Postmigration onset of disabling phobic disorders rarely occurs in isolation. That is, phobias usually coexist with other Axis I conditions (depression in particular, but sometimes other anxiety disorders, such as posttraumatic stress disorder or panic attacks). Axis II personality disorders are occasionally present. By the time these patients are encountered clinically, many are quite symptomatic and disabled. "Secondary gain" from the disorder may be present, such as requiring other family members to shop for the patient or drive the patient to work. These migrant patients have generally avoided readjustment or acculturation tasks as a result of their phobias. Self-relaxation, implosion, or cognitive desensitization tend to be less effective than social desensitization in these cases. Explanations for this include secondary gain issues, avoidance of social readjustment or acculturation, severity of symptoms, and unfamiliarity with (and lack of faith in) psychological modalities. Thus, a combination of pharmacotherapy (e.g., tricyclic, monoamine oxidase inhibitor, beta-blocking agent) and social desensitization is ordinarily necessary.

Social desensitization consists of repeated exposures to the noxious stimulus, initially in the company of others. These exposures may be begun after adequate medication to reduce the biophysiological concomitants of the panic-fear response. The presence of other people during desensitization serves two purposes: to motivate the patient toward exposure to the stimulus, which he or she avoids at all costs; and to enhance the development of interpersonal bonds, so that social-network reconstruction can ensue. Several people should be involved in the social desensitization, so that the patient does not become dependent on one or a few people to overcome the fear. Family members are especially prone to manipulation and "secondary gain," so they must be used sparingly and only after thorough education to the possible pitfalls. Neighbors, distant relatives, friends, fellow patients, and hospital or clinic staff can participate in this process. Initially patients will be most comfortable with those whom they rely upon and trust most. More than one person may also be reassuring. Eventually, patients should face the noxious stimulus with minimal support (e.g., one casual acquaintance). The next step consists of brief exposures to the stimulus while alone, then gradually building up the intensity and duration of the noxious stimulus (e.g., riding a bus, going to a funeral). Hospitalization or a day program may be necessary in severe cases.

Acculturation Therapy

Some foreign migrant patients have undergone little or no acculturation at the time that they enter treatment. Failure to acculturate even after years can be a factor in the genesis of their current disorder; or their disorder may have impeded their adjustment. Acculturation stress is apt to serve as a pathogenic factor in vulnerable, insecure, or inadequately prepared migrants (Szapocznik et al. 1978b, 1980). Migration can be described as a process of desocialization, with severe disorganization in the person's social and role system, to be followed by resocialization in the new environment. Full recovery from psychiatric disorders in foreign migrants who cannot return home (e.g., refugees, naturalized citizens) usually requires a level of acculturation that they have not yet attained.

Some migrant patients have already attained a reasonable level of acculturation, such as language skills, familiarity with the local community, and ability to travel and recreate locally. For these patients, individual one-to-one interventions may be adequate. These include coaching, education, support, suggestion, direction, and psychotherapies focused on the resistances or other psychological impediments to acculturation.

Some patients require more intensive and extensive acculturation therapies. Their psychological and social impediments are usually severe or long-lasting. Hospitalization or intensive outpatient programs may be needed to overcome these problems. Examples of problems associated with severe acculturation failure include the following: children and adults with learning disabilities, mental retardation, and organic brain damage; patients with a history of long-term residence in refugee camps, long-term welfare dependence, and/or long-term acculturation failure predating their psychiatric condition; substance-abusing (or other conduct-disordered) patients whose social networks are composed of similar persons; schizophrenic or bipolar patients who have not acculturated; and families with maladapting children, marital discord, or intergenerational stress, when these families are failing to acculturate (Szapocznik et al. 1978b; Szapocznik and Kurtines 1980).

Acculturation involves maintaining links to the past, as well as preparing for the future. Many people who fail in their acculturation tasks also have poor or tenuous ties to their own past. Enhanced ties to their own traditions can assist in preparing them to acquire parallel skills or knowledge in the new society, such as cooking, dancing, sports, and literacy. More secure in their ties to their cultural origins, they can become more free to explore a new culture (Ortiz and Arce 1984).

In a context of migration, the "traditional" culture of course changes, as it is reassessed and renegotiated. Some traditional elements are abandoned, some kept and strengthened, others kept but altered. Foreigners thus have to adapt to their own changing expatriate communities, since these are not a mirror image of the society that was left behind. Since migrants themselves are a biased sample, their expatriate communities can be expected to be a biased reflection of the old society. The surrounding society also works changes among the expatriates, at times in unpredictable ways. Immigrants may thus need to be not just bicultural (i.e, acculturated to the previous culture and the new society) but tricultural (i.e., acculturated to the old, the new, and the changing expatriate cultures).

Acculturation cuts across virtually all phases of daily life, as well as across the life cycle (Chance 1965; Mann 1958; Richman et al. 1987). Life areas as well as goals and attitudes to be addressed in acculturation therapy include the following:

Life Area	Goals and Activities
Technology and related skills	Driver's license, home repair, use of modern appliances
Values, customs, symbols, attitudes	Folktales, literature, cinema, theatre, television, art, music, history
Language, nonverbal communication	English as a Second Language courses, Sesame Street television programs
Recreation, avocations, hobbies	Sports events, family outings and pastimes, age-appropriate activities
Rituals, celebrations, festivals	Participating with native persons in local events, and with the expatriate community in traditional events
Occupational skills, employment	Vocational counseling, occupational and industrial therapy, education, training, job-seeking and job-application skills
Transportation, communication	Use of local and national transportation, mail, telephone, parcel post
Family life, life cycle	Childbirth, child rearing, marriage and divorce laws, funeral practices, inheritance laws
Security, legal system	Self-protection, home security, dangerous times and places and behaviors, police services, law enforcement, laws, use of attorneys, court system, jail, prison, commitment laws
Education and training systems	Levels of education, certification, licensure, continuing education, on-the-job training
Social agencies and resources	Private and public, religious and secular, ethnic and nonethnic

Life Area	*Goals and Activities*
Health systems	Generalist and specialist, public and private, common causes of morbidity and mortality, preventing illness, use of the health care system
Informed citizen participation (or noncitizen observation)	Newspaper, radio and television news programs, modern history, current events discussions, political science, American studies, economic situation, prices.

Younger migrants tend to acculturate more readily than older migrants, whether the migration is within a country (Richman et al. 1987) or from one country to another (Krupinski and Burrows 1986). Thus, special acculturation therapies are most apt to be needed for adult migrants, rather than children. However, even children and adolescent migrant patients can experience role stress, acculturation problems, and identity confusion (Naditch and Morrissey 1976). Youthful migrants are at risk if the usual acculturation experiences (e.g., in school, neighborhood) are not feasible or likely to occur, or if the family does not provide a secure environment to permit concurrent individual and family change.

Resocialization Therapy

Some migrants have spent months, years, or even decades in artificial, confined, or dependent settings that can undermine psychosocial skills and social competency. This group includes migrants from certain Indian reservations and ghetto neighborhoods with "welfare subcultures," refugee camps, prisoner-of-war camps, concentration camps, and torture prisons, and migrants who have been incarcerated as hostages. Prolonged exposure in these settings is apt—in vulnerable persons—to produce "learned helplessness," dependency, passive aggressiveness, fatalism, a sense of entitlement, and ingratitude to

219

assistance. First described by the Swiss psychiatrist Pfister-Ammende (1973) among refugees after World War II, this phenomenon of learned helplessness has since been observed in a variety of oppressed and victimized persons. Manifestations of social maladjustment include a robotlike way of relating to others, social and family violence, the formation of an antiauthority subculture outside the societal mainstream, and the perpetuation of a large number of people subject to decompensation with minimal stresses (Chan and Loveridge 1987).

This desocialized condition can be replicated by reproducing or continuing the person's dependency and disability. Such morbidity-producing strategies include prolonged welfare payments, social security for people of preretirement age, veteran's payments requiring disability behavior, and lengthy hospitalization. These disabling strategies re-expose people to conditions in which nothing that they do has any effect (Yager 1975). Thus, the system induces them to remain helpless and to complain interminably. Resocialization strategies include the following:

- Providing meaningful work, with the opportunity for training and advancement;
- Facilitating community organization, with the opportunity to have some influence over organization and events;
- Associating with groups that can assign identity, role, and prestige; and
- Increasing general awareness regarding the desocializing effects of certain experiences (e.g., concentration camps, warfare, welfare) on many people, the dangers of a "chronic victim" identity, and the means for extricating oneself, one's family, and one's peers from this morbid condition.

Hospitalization

Due to absence of a family, some migrants who might otherwise be treated at home must be hospitalized. This group includes some students away from home, military inductees, and tourists. Diagnostic dilemmas, the likelihood of organic factors, and communication problems may prompt hospitalization for assessment purposes. Treatment in a secure, monitored place is indicated for migrants dangerous to others (especially paranoid patients), dangerous to self (especially depressed or "homesick" patients), unable to adhere to treatment (perhaps due to limited knowledge), or unwilling to comply with treatment (due to complexity of the regimen, unfamiliarity with home treatment regimens). Numerous "treatment failure" patients with depression, mania, schizophrenia, disabling anxiety disorders, and paranoia respond rapidly to treatment once it is applied and monitored in a hospital setting. For less sophisticated patients and families, hospitalization can subvert frenetic dashes hither and yon seeking fantasied "cures."

Hospital treatment can serve particular therapeutic ends for migrant patients. As described above, social desensitization of phobias can be initiated. Refugees and other foreign migrants, fearful of local people, have the opportunity to replace their stereotypes with personal experiences, achieved through contacts with other patients and staff. Patients can begin acculturation therapy through community meetings, group therapy, family sessions, occupational therapy, recreational activities, and off-ward forays. For family members immersed in their own readjustment and acculturation, hospitalization of a disturbed and disturbing family member can provide much needed respite, followed by renewed commitment to the patient's wellbeing (Geiser et al. 1988).

Hospitalization can also pose several disadvantages for migrant patients, especially those from markedly different societies. Unfamiliarity with English can exacerbate the patient's sense of isolation, especially if other patients and staff do not speak the patient's language. Patients may not want to eat the local hospital fare and, as a result, may experience weight loss or may demand that family members bring food. Separation from family members may be a great burden not only for the patient but also for the family. Some families may feel obligated to provide around-the-clock attention by family "sitters"—a common custom in many countries, where family members provide virtually all nursing services in the hospital, other than special observations and treatments. Sociocultural isolation can be heightened further if the patient is the sole representative of his or her culture on the ward.

Nursing staff may experience initial frustration in caring for patients from different cultures or patients who speak no English. Nurses may state that it is impossible for them to care for someone unless they and the patient speak a common language. With education and experience, these staff resistances can be overcome. Nurses, like psychiatrists, need daily access to translators in order to conduct reassessments, educate the inpatient, and negotiate day-to-day living arrangements. Behavior modification programs can be salutory for staff and patients, since these methods depend primarily on behavior rather than language. Medication routines and vital sign observations can usually be arranged without difficulty. Exposure to community meetings, recreational activities, exercise, group meals, walks, and occupational therapy serve two purposes: assessment, to see how the patient manages these experiences; and treatment, to facilitate the patient's comfort in and adjustment to the new environment. As patients improve clinically, their language facility and social skills often develop also.

Intensive Outpatient Programs

Day, evening, and weekend programs can provide most of the advantages of hospitalization, while possessing few of the disadvantages. Patients can eat their morning and evening meals with their families, sleep at home, and not experience unremitting cultural isolation and separation from family. At the same time, it is possible to monitor vital signs, administer medications, assess the patient's treatment response, initiate vigorous acculturation therapy, and provide the family with some respite. This can be accomplished at a weekly cost of about one-third to one-fourth that of inpatient hospitalization. Availability of such programs can lead to a reduction of inpatient length of stay, at times avoiding hospital inpatient admissions altogether.

Migrant and nonmigrant patients in day programs can benefit one another in several ways. Nonmigrants can provide social "practice" for migrant patients engaged in acculturation. Migrant patients can add to the cultural diversity and richness of the program, thereby undermining ethnic bias and racial prejudice. The presence of migrants can help local patients (and staff) become more aware of their own society and its cultural heritages.

As with inpatient staff, staff in day programs may be initially overwhelmed by patients from unfamiliar cultures or patients who do not speak English well. Hiring staff from cultures representing the patient population is an effective step in overcoming these resistances and biases. Language problems loom largest for group therapy and community meetings; are intermediate for education, social-skills-building sessions (which can be videotaped), and group projects; and are least for exercise-movement therapy, art-music therapy, recreation therapy, occupational therapy, and industrial therapy. English language and/or acculturation training can be designed to meet the special needs of migrant patients.

Milieu Changes

Foster home placement of children presents special challenges in a multiracial, multiethnic society (Redick and Wood 1982; Westermeyer 1977). Insofar as possible, children requiring foster homes should be placed with families who possess the same racial and ethnic characteristics of the patient. Failure to do so can add to the obstacles that migrant children and adolescents must overcome, since it is difficult enough to adjust to a new home and community, without also having to adjust to a new culture or language. In leaving refugee camps, adolescent refugees also lose peer support—an important source

223

of support for this group (Looney 1979). In a society like the United States, unaccompanied refugee children and racial minority children are apt to be placed in Caucasian homes. This usually leads to problems of racial-ethnic discontinuity (Westermeyer 1979a, 1979b), variously described as the apple (red Indian outside, white inside), banana (Asian outside, white inside), or Oreo-cookie (black outside, white inside) syndrome. This phenomenon is characterized by the following: eventual rejection by the majority white society, during middle to late adolescence due to racial bias; failure in the minority racial group due to inability to function psychologically and socially in that group during late adolescence and young adulthood; identity confusion, loss of self-esteem, alienation from adoptive parents, self-hate, self-destructive behaviors; and increased risk to school drop out, underachievement, problems relating to authority, divorce, and/or employment difficulties.

Foster placement can involve other risks as well. Foster children with serious mental health problems can produce severe stresses on families and marriages. Other children in the family may be neglected; divorce can ensue even in families that were functioning adequately prior to placement of the child. Family guidance and counseling for foster families caring for disturbed or disturbing children is warranted. Lower-class families are apt to assume the care of foster children in order to garner extra income and, especially in rural areas, to benefit from their labor, thus resulting in poor ensocialization experiences. Egan (1985), in a study of 27 unaccompanied Vietnamese minors in American foster homes, observed "satisfactory" family adjustment in 9 cases, "inadequate" family function but with some minimal adaptation in 13 cases, and "perilous" outcomes in families with dysfunction in 5 cases. Fully two-thirds of these foster children were showing family adjustment that was inadequate or worse. Sexual and physical abuse in foster homes are unfortunately not rare, especially in solo parent homes whether led by a male or female (Williams and Westermeyer 1983).

Foster placement is sometimes needed for migrant children and adolescents living in intact or partial families (Chan and Loveridge 1987). This alternative is especially common in solo-parent families or families in which one or both parents are substance abusers or chronically mentally ill. The children usually manifest substance abuse, school failure, truancy, family violence, or violence at school. Foster placement for 1 or 2 years, during which parents and child receive treatment, can be effective, permitting reestablishment of the family unit. Families in which a temporary period of foster placement proved beneficial include the following:

- A 28-year-old divorced alcoholic mother, American Indian, with two children; eldest (11-year-old) son was abusing volatile inhalants and being truant from school;
- A 36-year-old widowed Lao refugee, mother of six children, who had a major melancholic depression; eldest (16-year-old) son and a 15-year-old son were abusing cannabis daily, stealing from their mother, and threatening their mother with physical violence;
- A 32-year-old Eastern European Jewish widow, disabled with major depression; 12-year-old son was abusing a variety of street drugs and was fighting at school.

Adopted children among nonmigrants are at higher risk to psychopathology, and this probably applies as well to migrant adopted children. Behavioral and emotional problems (e.g., nightmares, tantrums, fearfulness), occur frequently after placement (Sokoloff et al. 1984). Adoptive parents may have difficulty understanding the behavior (normal or abnormal) of the recently arrived adoptee from a different culture (Wolters 1980). At least during childhood, these adopted children appear to do well in the years following stable placement (McBogg and Wouri 1979). Problems in those adopted children with racial-ethnic discontinuity generally begin during adolescence and early adulthood (Westermeyer 1979b; Williams and Westermeyer 1983). Common problems consist of substance abuse, runaway, delinquent behavior, suicide attempts, and depression.

Halfway-house placement and residential treatment pose many of the problems of hospitalization for migrants, especially those from markedly different societies. Still, certain advantages can be realized. Migrants can acculturate more readily there than at home in many cases. Cost is less than in a hospital. If a few or several residents share race and ethnicity with the patient, they can form their own expatriate subgroup. Such a subgroup can then warrant the hiring of a staff member from that ethnic group. Several advantages associated with hospitalization may occur in these settings, including observation of vital signs, supervised medication, reporting changes in patient's condition, and respite for the acculturating family. Important risks include exposure to the dangers of the community, i.e., substance abuse, assault, robbery, rape (all of which we have encountered among our patients in these settings, usually located in dangerous sections of town).

Shelters can be helpful for migrants exposed to the threat of physical abuse at home. Adult migrants failing at readjustment may displace their self-hate and impose their rage upon family members, including elderly parents, spouses, and children. Most shelters are willing to accept migrants temporarily, even those unable to speak English (assuming that a translator can assist).

Returning home to the community of origin can be therapeutic for some migrants. In doing so, they may be able to reduce their stresses (e.g., for new social networks, language) while increasing access to resources (e.g., family, old friend). This is especially true for those who have relocated alone for education, training, military service, or work. The disadvantage of this alternative is that it conveys a failure experience—i.e., that the person has been unable to succeed at a significant new venture. Ordinarily it is best to attempt treatment in situ, aimed at helping the person to adjust, and keeping the return home as an alternative of last resort. Generally the decision to return home is made on various grounds: the patient's and the family's wishes, insurance or financial ability to pay for care in the United States, visa regulations, and immigration law. In the face of a deteriorating course or poor response to treatment, a return home should be recommended.

Some migrants cannot be obliged to return home, such as immigrants, naturalized citizens, or refugees—even though a trial at home might be warranted on clinical grounds. Refugees may not be able to return home safely. Some immigrants and naturalized citizens may not have the resources to return home, even if they wanted to do so. Under the circumstances, the one alternative is to try and enhance the patient's acculturation.

References

Berne E: Transactional Analysis in Psychotherapy. New York, Grove Press, 1961

Brower IC: Counseling Vietnamese. Personnel Guidance Journal 58:646–652, 1980

Chance NA: Acculturation, self-identification and personal adjustment. American Anthropologist 67:372–393, 1965

Chan KB, Loveridge D: Refugees "in transit": Vietnamese in a refugee camp in Hong Kong. International Migration Review 21:745–759, 1987

Egan MG: A family assessment challenge: refugee youth and foster family adaptation. Topics in Clinical Nursing 7:64–69, 1985

Geiser R, Hoche L, King J: Respite care for mentally ill patients and their families. Hosp Community Psychiatry 39:291–295, 1988

Kaslow FW (ed): The International Book of Family Therapy. New York, Brunner/Mazel, 1982

Kim SC: Family therapy for Asian Americans: a strategic-structural framework. Psychotherapy 22:342–348, 1985

Krupinski J, Burrows G (eds): The Price of Freedom: Young

Indochinese Refugees in Australia. New York, Pergamon, 1986

Lappin J, Scott S: Intervention in a Vietnamese refugee family, in Ethnicity and Family Therapy. Edited by McGoldrich M, Pearce JK, Giordano J. New York, Guilford, 1982, pp 483–491

Looney JG: Adolescents as refugees. Adolesc Psychiatry 7:199–208, 1979

Mann JW: Group relations and the marginal man. Human Relations 11:77–92, 1958

Marmar CR, Horowitz MJ, Weiss DS, et al: A controlled trial of brief psychotherapy and mutual-help group treatment of conjugal bereavement. Am J Psychiatry 145:203–209, 1988

Masters R, Friedman LN, Getzel G: Helping families of homicide victims: a multidimensional approach. Journal of Traumatic Stress 1:109–125, 1988

McBogg P, Wouri D: Outcome of adopted Vietnamese children. Clin Pediatr 18:179–183, 1979

McGoldrich M, Pearce JK, Giordano J (eds): Ethnicity and Family Therapy. New York, Guilford, 1982

Naditch MD, Morrissey RF: Role stress, personality, and psychopathology in a group of immigrant adolescents. J Abnorm Psychol 85:113–118, 1976

Ortiz V, Arce CH: Language orientation and mental health status among persons of Mexican descent. Hispanic Journal of Behavioral Sciences 6:127–143, 1984

Pfister-Ammende M: Mental hygiene in refugee camps, in Uprooting and After. Edited by Zwingmann C, Pfister-Ammende M. New York, Springer-Verlag, 1973, pp 241–251

Redick LT, Wood B: Cross-cultural problems for Southeast Asian refugee minors. Child Welfare 61:365–373, 1982

Richman JA, Gaviria M, Flaherty J, et al: The process of acculturation: theoretical perspectives and an empirical investigation in Peru. Soc Sci Med 25:839–847, 1987

Sokoloff B, Carlin J, Pham H: Five-year follow-up of Vietnamese refugee children in the United States. Clin Pediatr 10:565–570, 1984

Speck RV, Attneave CL: Family Networks. New York, Pantheon, 1973

Szapocznik J, Kurtines W: Acculturation, biculturalism and adjustment among Cuban Americans, in Psychological Dimensions on the Acculturation Process: Theory, Models and Some New Findings. Edited by Padilla A. Boulder, CO, Westview, 1980, pp 139–159

Szapocznik J, Daruna P, Scopetta MA, et al: The characteristics of Cuban immigrant inhaler abusers. Am J Drug Alcohol Abuse 4:377–390, 1978a

Szapocznik J, Scopetta MA, Arandale MA, et al: Cuban value structure: clinical implications. J Consult Clin Psychol 46:961–970, 1978b

Szapocznik J, Kurtines W, Fernandez T: Biculturalism involvement and adjustment in Hispanic-American youths. International Journal of Intercultural Relations 4:353–365, 1980

Szapocznik J, Santisteban D, Kurtines W, et al: Bicultural effectiveness training: a treatment intervention for enhancing intercultural adjustment in Cuban American families. Hispanic Journal of Behavioral Sciences 6:317–344, 1984

Tseng WS: Cultural aspects of family assessment. International Journal of Family Psychiatry 6:19–31, 1985

Westermeyer J: Cross-racial foster home placement among Native American psychiatric patients. J Natl Med Assoc 69:231–236, 1977

Westermeyer J: Ethnic identity problems among 10 Indian psychiatric patients. Int J Soc Psychiatry 25:188–197, 1979a

Westermeyer J: The "apple" syndrome: the effects of racial-ethnic discontinuity. Journal of Operational Psychiatry 10:134–140, 1979b

Williams C, Westermeyer J: Problems among adolescent Southeast Asian refugees: a descriptive study. J Nerv Ment Dis 171:79–85, 1983

Wolters WHG: Psychosocial problems in young foreign adopted children. Acta Paedopsychiatrica 46:67–81, 1980

Yager J: What happens when nothing you do matters? Contemporary Psychology 20:921–922, 1975